THE BOBBS-MERRILL STUDIES IN SOCIOLOGY

The Exploitation of Illness in Capitalist Society

Howard Waitzkin
and
Barbara Waterman

BOBBS-MERRILL EDUCATIONAL PUBLISHING
INDIANAPOLIS

To Simone

The Bobbs-Merrill Company, Inc.
4300 West 62nd Street
Indianapolis, Indiana 46268

First Edition
Fourth Printing—1977

Library of Congress Cataloging in Publication Data
Waitzkin, Howard and Waterman, Barbara
The exploitation of illness in capitalist society
(The Bobbs-Merrill studies in sociology)
Bibliography: p.
1. Social medicine. 2. Medical care—United
States. I. Waterman, Barbara, joint author.
II. Title [DNLM: 1. Delivery of health care.—
U. S. 2. Medicine—U. S. 3. Politics—U. S.
4. Sociology—U. S. WB50 AA1 W2e 1974]
RA418.W34 362.1'04'220973 73-19706
ISBN 0-672-61327-1 (pbk.)

The Exploitation of Illness in Capitalist Society

Preface

It seems appropriate in this preface to offer a few comments about our own value assumptions and personal commitments in social research.* Social scientists concerned with health and illness encounter human suffering as part of their daily work. There are various possible responses to the encounter with suffering. One approach involves a psychic compartmentalization of the intellectual problems which suffering raises. Those who adopt this approach present empirical observations and theoretical analyses without explicit reference to the pain they have witnessed and probably have shared.

A second response to suffering extends the scope of social scientific work to include the "policy implications" of research findings. Statements of policy implications, usually appended at the conclusion of research reports, tend to exhort those in power to make certain specified reforms, but without basic changes in present institutional structures.

A third approach calls for radical criticism of existing social institutions, as well as political activism, directed toward basic institutional change. Gouldner offers a detailed exposition of this latter approach:

> The extrication of the liberative potential of Academic Sociology, no less than that of historical Marxism, is not to be accomplished by research alone. It will also require action and criticism, efforts to change the social world and efforts to change social science, both of which are profoundly interconnected, if for no other reason than that social science is a **part** of the social world as well as a **conception** of it (1970:13).

From this perspective, radical criticism comprises an appropriate and desirable part of social research and analysis. Our own observations of the relationships between illness and social structure have led us to adopt the third approach as the most tenable personally.

This short book presents a critical analysis of existing institutional structures in the American health system, as well as an appraisal of theory in medical sociology. In the introductory section we consider medicine as a social institution and the sociopolitical context of illness. In Section 2, after discussing previous theoretical positions in medical sociology, we outline an alternative theoretical approach. Section 3 attempts to show that the sick role, by providing a controllable form of deviance,

---

* The preface is based in part on excerpts from "Health and the Family: A Review Essay," by Howard Waitzkin, in Social Science and Medicine 7(1973):387–394. Reprinted courtesy of Pergamon Press.

mitigates potential conflicts in such institutions as prisons, the armed forces, and the Selective Service System; by helping prevent conflicts, the sick role reduces the probability of basic institutional change. Stratification in medicine is the topic of Section 4; the control of information is studied as a major source of medical stratification. In Section 5 we analyze the problem of empire building in American medicine, with emphasis on the major proposed reforms in the health system—national health insurance and health maintenance organizations. The study concludes with a brief discussion of the relationships between improved health care and broad sociopolitical change.

Criticism of the present system, of course, is not enough. The social scientist interested in changing social institutions also should offer a positive program. Although we outline in the concluding chapter several programmatic requirements for a humanistic, nonexploiting health system, a detailed exposition of new structural arrangements to care for the sick is beyond the scope of this study. We might emphasize, however, our general agreement with George Bernard Shaw: "The social solution of the medical problem depends on that large, slowly advancing, pettishly resisted integration of society called generally Socialism" (1963:67).

Several teachers have stimulated the development of our ideas, by forcing us to think analytically about new problems and by offering their criticisms and encouragement. Talcott Parsons, Renée C. Fox, S. F. Sampson, Elliot G. Mishler, Stanley King, and Odin W. Anderson have provided models of rigorous sociological thinking, while always encouraging us to formulate our own unique approaches. Loring Conant, Jr., John Stoeckle, Roger Sweet, and Charles Lewis have demonstrated the practice of humane clinical medicine, worthy of emulation. Members of the Medical Committee for Human Rights, Health Policy Advisory Center, Student Health Organization, Medical Resistance Union, and Roxbury Tenants of Harvard Association have helped develop our ideas concerning the political ramifications of health care. Hermann Lisco, Myron Sharaf, and Thomas Sisson have overcome innumerable obstacles to conducting sociological and medical work at the same time.

Financial support from the Popper Foundation, Roothbert Fund, Rosenthal Foundation, and Johnson Foundation facilitated the preparation of this book. We also thank Halsted Holman, Bonnie Obrig, and the Clinical Scholars Program at Stanford University for assistance with the manuscript. Finally, Eliot Freidson provided a very useful critique of our work.

1 Introduction: The Sociopolitical Context of Medicine

Is a humane health care system possible in a capitalist society?

Norman Bethune, a Canadian physician who served the forces of Mao

Tse-tung during the War of Resistance against Japan, described the wounds of Chinese soldiers and traced their cause to capitalism:

> *Wounds like little dried pools, caked with black-brown earth; wounds with torn edges frilled with black gangrene. . . .*
>
> *Is it possible that a few rich men, a small class of men, have persuaded a million poor men to attack, and attempt to destroy, another million men as poor as they? So that the rich may be richer still? Behind the army stand the militarists. Behind the militarists stand finance capital and the capitalist. Brothers in blood; companions in crime.*
>
> *What do these enemies of the human race look like? . . . They are honoured. They call themselves, and are called, gentlemen. What a travesty of the name! Gentlemen! They are the pillars of the State, of the church, of society. They support private and public charity out of the excess of their wealth. They endow institutions. In their private lives they are kind and considerate. They obey the law, their law, the law of property. But there is one sign by which these gentle gunmen can be told. Threaten a reduction in the profit of their money and the beast in them awakes with a snarl. They become as ruthless as savages, brutal as madmen, remorseless as executioners. Such men as these must perish if the human race is to continue. There can be no permanent peace in the world while they live. Such an organization of human society as permits them to exist must be abolished.*
>
> *These men make the wounds (1969: 184–186).*

In war, the relationships between social structure and illness are starkly evident. Bethune analyzed the imperialist ventures by which Japanese capitalism created the suffering of poor Japanese and Chinese soldiers (Mao Tse-tung, 1961). In "peace," the interconnections between suffering and social structure are somewhat subtler. Under capitalism, illness comes to be viewed as a source of profit and power—for the medical profession, for corporations which produce drugs and equipment, and for hospitals and other organizations which provide health care. In this book we are concerned with the exploitation of suffering and the forms of social organization which foster this exploitation.

MEDICINE AS A SOCIAL INSTITUTION

To start, some definitions are appropriate. *Illness* involves pathophysiologic processes in individual patients. *Medicine,* on the other hand, is a social institution. By this we mean the following. Definitions of health and illness are not constant but vary in different sociocultural milieus. For example, American definitions differ from those of other cultures, and this variability gives rise to conflicts when Western medicine—often patterned along the American model—is introduced in competition with established indigenous traditions (Parsons, 1972; Saunders, 1954; Shiloh, 1968). Most societies have developed a number of *roles* related to health and illness, for example the roles of nurse, doctor, patient, hospital administrator, orderly, etc. The *role-expectations* (the ways in which people who occupy these roles are expected to act) associated with medical roles pattern the behavior of healers and the sick in predictable ways. The totality of roles and role-expectations related to health and illness comprises the *institution of medicine* (cf. Parsons, 1951:39).

This definition of the institution of medicine is intentionally a broad one. The institution of medicine includes a large number of collectivities, which are systems of "concretely interactive specific roles" (Parsons, 1951:39). Typical collectivities within the institution include the doctor-patient, doctor-nurse, and doctor-doctor relationships, as well as larger aggregates—for example, professional organizations of physicians, hospitals, and pharmaceutical companies (Parsons, 1970:337–342). Because the definition is conceived in the broadest possible terms, other examples of role patterns within the institution of medicine include familial relationships, such as mother—sick child, and occupational relationships, such as employer—sick employee. "Medicine as a social institution" refers to all these diverse role patterns related to health and illness.

THE SOCIOPOLITICAL CONTEXT OF MEDICINE AND THE MEDICOCIVIL STRUCTURE

Medicine and the polity: health care under capitalist and socialist political systems The sick do not suffer in isolation from the broad sociopolitical structures of the societies in which they live. There are numerous interconnections between medicine and the broader social system of which medicine is a part (cf. Alford, 1972; Kelman, 1971; Lichtman, 1971). In all societies, health care is a service provided by one group of people (health workers) to another (patients). Societies differ greatly, however, in the ways they organize this service. The organizational forms which govern the treatment of the sick reflect broad normative principles within a society; the normative framework within which health workers and patients interact may be called the society's *medicocivil structure.*

The medicocivil structure of a society is intimately tied to the set of rights and responsibilities encompassed by the notion of citizenship. It has been said, for example, that with the transition to modernity, certain rights emerged which by consensus came to be held by all citizens. These rights included the right of education, the right of participation in the legislative process through the franchise, and the rights of free association and combination into voluntary organizations (Bendix, 1969).

Is health care also a basic right of all citizens? Capitalist societies have shown a certain ambiguity on this point. During the industrializing period of capitalism (the late nineteenth and early twentieth centuries), the health of individual workers was subordinated to the productivity sought by capitalists. The consequent ill health and early death of industrial workers during this period has been amply documented (Rosen, 1958). Unionization, in addition to its goal of economic well-being, was motivated largely by the attempt to improve those conditions of work which created illness and physical suffering (Merrium, 1971). The enactment of legislation regulating safety standards and working conditions represented not only a political response to unions' demands, but also an implicit recognition of the workers' right to good health.

The ambiguity of patients' right to health care also has been reflected in the principle of a "sliding scale" for physicians' fees. In private practice, individual physicians have been able to charge the highest fee which the traffic would bear, under the single constraint that a high price would not severely reduce the demand for their services. Generally the price which physicians could command has been viewed as one mark of their competence and reputation. On the other hand, when patients cannot afford to pay a physician's price, the principle of the sliding scale has called for a downward adjustment of fee, to correspond with patients' financial resources (Parsons, 1970:341–342).

It should be noted that the sliding scale depends mainly on patients' initiative in pleading poverty; many patients avoid protestation of need by simply refraining from seeking medical care. In addition, the sliding scale allows great discretion for the physician, who autonomously can select those patients for whom the scale is applicable and can then determine a patient's position on the scale according to unspecified criteria. The assumption also has been that all patients must pay some fee, however small. The rationale usually offered is that patients' serious commitment to the doctor-patient relationship and their reliable compliance with the doctor's advice are enhanced by the payment of a fee.

While the sliding scale has not prevented a maldistribution of health services favoring wealthy patients, its existence implies that all patients have some right to health services. If patients are unabashed about admitting indigence and aggressive in seeking care, the sliding scale recognizes the physician's responsibility to give attention to patients who cannot afford standard fees.

Despite less dangerous working conditions in many industries, the tension between profit and good health in capitalist societies has persisted; the sliding scale has not solved the health problems of the poor. Capitalists never lack ingenuity in discovering sources of profit. Recently they have found increasing profit in illness. In this sense the tension between profit and health extends beyond the conditions of work which engender illness. Rather, health care becomes a commodity to be bought and sold like other goods and services.

Profit from health care accrues both to individual physicians and to the growing industries which provide health services and produce medical products. On the individual level, physicians have maintained the highest level of income among the professions (Table 1). As public and private expenditures for health care have increased since the advent of Medicare and Medicaid, physicians' incomes have risen to even higher levels (Figures 1, 2; cf. Marmor, 1968).

9

Table 1. Median annual income by profession, 1970–1971

Profession	Income ($)*
Physicians	41,500
Attorneys	21,396
Accountants	19,800
Engineers	17,880
Professors	16,799
Teachers	9,269

* Net income, indicates income after deduction of expenses related to professional activities.

Sources: U.S., Department of Commerce, 1972:68, 122,131; U.S., Department of Labor, 1972:16–17.

Typically, a small proportion of physicians file the largest number of claims for payment under government insurance programs and receive the greatest total reimbursement (Lewis and Keairnes, 1970). Because of often exorbitant payments, these doctors attract criticism to government spending for health care. Despite initial opposition to government insur-

Figure 1. National Health Expenditures, United States, 1955–1970

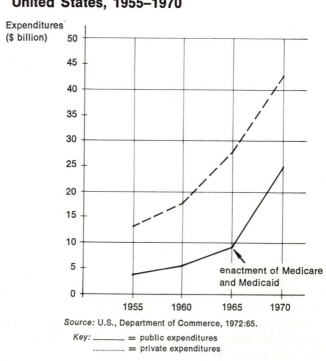

Source: U.S., Department of Commerce, 1972:65.

Key: _____ = public expenditures
.... = private expenditures

Figure 2. Physicians' median net income from practice, 1959 and 1965–1970

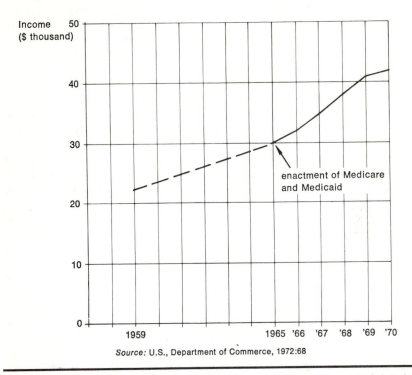

Source: U.S., Department of Commerce, 1972:68

ance programs, physicians have come to understand the financial gains potentially available under these programs. Thus, although a majority of physicians initially objected to Medicare, attitudes quickly changed after legislation was enacted; approximately 81 percent of doctors in practice ultimately favored significant federal spending for medical care (Colombotos, 1969).

The price of medical services, unlike other goods and services, is not subject to the usual constraints of supply and demand. More than in other professions, the supply of physicians is sharply limited. Restricted access to the profession occurs at two stages: acceptance to medical school and licensure to practice. The American Medical Association consistently has opposed the federal financial assistance necessary for the establishment of new medical schools and for expanding the number of available positions for students. As a result of the restriction of positions, over 7,000 qualified college graduates who have completed premedical requirements annually are denied acceptance at medical schools (American Medical News, 1971; Dube et al., 1971).

Acceptance criteria in the United States, unlike those in socialist countries, are based largely on subjective characteristics rather than academic achievement per se. That is, American medical schools' admission policies often reflect a fadism which partly derives from public pressures (to favor minority groups, women, and so on) and partly depends on personal preferences of individuals in key positions on admissions committees. In contrast, acceptance to medical school in socialist countries generally depends on the completion of specific academic prerequisites, and is thus based on more objective and consistent criteria, rather than on cultural trends or personal whims.

Examinations for licensure and specialty certification further limit access to the medical profession. It has been forcefully argued that extensive licensure provisions, while scarcely assuring minimal standards of competence within the profession, seriously reduce the supply of physicians (Friedman, 1962:149–160).

Moreover, physicians themselves can directly affect the demand for their services. In general, patients rely on their doctors' advice in deciding the frequency of their appointments. Physicians also enhance the demand for their colleagues' services by advising referrals and consultations, which patients usually feel bound to pursue. These sources of "derived demand"—that is, demand directly created by the producers of health services—increase the profits available for individual physicians (Feldstein, 1966).

In capitalist society, the view of health care as a commodity and source of profit has extended beyond individual medical practitioners themselves. Increasingly, illness has brought profits to large American corporations. The most obvious example of profit from illness is the pharmaceutical industry, whose drug sales presently total over $7 billion per year and are increasing at a rate of about 9 percent annually. The pharmaceutical industry spends approximately 25 percent of its income from sales on advertising and promotion, including gifts to doctors and medical students which are intended to influence physicians' prescribing habits. Other rapidly growing industries include companies producing hospital supplies and equipment, whose profits climbed 15 to 25 percent after the enactment of Medicare legislation in 1965, and the private nursing home corporations, which have created a multibillion dollar enterprise expanding rapidly with the availability of federal funds for elderly patients (Ehrenreich and Ehrenreich, 1969; Health Policy Advisory Center, 1970:95–123).

Despite ambiguities reflected in occupational safety legislation and the sliding fee scale, capitalist societies have tended to permit the financial exploitation of illness. When health is viewed as a commodity with a price, it tends to be differentially distributed among members of a society. As a variety of studies have documented, low-income people have inadequate access to medical services and facilities, as compared to wealthier patients (e.g., Koos, 1967; Strauss, 1972; Kosa et al., 1969).

In fact, the unequal distribution of medical care is one characteristic by which a population is stratified. As Miller and Roby have pointed out, the maldistribution of health services bears a complex relationship to income. Patients with a low level of income obviously cannot purchase health services and related goods such as medications as easily as higher-income patients. Moreover, health care in capitalist societies increasingly is offered as a fringe benefit of employment. Employers receive tax advantages by providing health benefits rather than increasing wages, since the former are not subject to Social Security or similar taxes. Nonmonetary compensation such as health care ultimately increases the inequalities between the many poor unorganized workers who do not receive fringe benefits and the rest of the labor force (Miller and Roby, 1970:52–56).

In addition to the "vertical" maldistribution of medical services based on income, "horizontal" maldistribution, deriving from geographical discrepancies in facilities and personnel, also occurs under capitalist medical systems. In the United States, for example, extreme shortages of physicians are experienced in rural areas like Appalachia and the Great Plains states, as well as in urban districts with predominantly black and Spanish-speaking populations. On the other hand, more affluent parts of cities and suburbs on the East Coast and West Coast have large concentrations of medical personnel (Fein, 1967). The presence of large medical centers, as well as financial and cultural advantages in these areas, inhibits physicians from practicing where there is the greatest actual need for their services.

Countries with socialist political systems vary in their administrative arrangements to care for the sick. As we discuss later, certain socialist nations have been more successful than others in meeting the health needs of the population. These countries differ also in the extent to which they permit individual physicians to engage in private practice and to receive direct monetary payment from patients. Explicitly or implicitly, however, most socialist regimes espouse two basic principles as part of the medicocivil structure.

First, *health care is a right of all citizens.* Health care thus assumes a position essentially equivalent to public education, since it represents a service to which all members of a society are entitled by virtue of citizenship.

The general principle of health care as a right implies two corollaries. In the first place, any financial impediments restricting the individual patient's access to health services must be removed. This means that physicians are paid directly by some arm of the government for services provided to low-income patients, or that the government reimburses patients for payments they make to physicians. In most socialist nations, doctors are employees of a national health service, obtain a salary from government revenues, and receive either no or nominal fees from individual patients. An alternative arrangement depends on a system of national health insurance, under which doctors are paid by the government on a fee-for-service basis or patients pay the usual fee to doctors and later obtain reimbursement from the government (W. Glaser, 1970).

A second corollary of health care as a right pertains to the problem of distribution: any maldistribution of health personnel and facilities which limits patients' ability to obtain needed services must be rectified. Thus, the country tries to bring medical workers, hospitals, and clinics to rural areas and to parts of cities which previously have had shortages of facilities and inadequate staffing. Socialist countries have used a number of methods in their attempts to correct geographical maldistribution. One method provides extra financial incentives, through higher salaries, to physicians who agree to serve in rural areas. Since this technique remains essentially voluntary in nature, physicians may choose to remain in cities despite the available financial incentives, and the problem of maldistribution may persist to a greater or lesser degree. Another method to overcome geographical inequalities involves compulsory measures, which require medical workers to serve for a specified tenure of duty in needy areas of a country. Although compulsory redistribution has achieved great improvements in several socialist countries, motivational problems have remained, leading to a rapid turnover rate of personnel serving rural patients. Alternatively, a country may try to correct maldistribution by training a corps of paramedical workers, who perform most functions of physicians but refer difficult diagnostic or therapeutic problems to urban centers. This latter approach has been especially successful in large socialist countries with remote villages such as the People's Republic of China. (The distinction between national health service and national health insurance is elaborated in Section 5; the techniques employed in the correction of distributional inequalities are considered in greater detail in Section 6).

A second basic principle governing health care in socialist countries is that *illness should not be exploited for profit.* In a sense, this principle is tied to a more general dictum concerning profit. According to Marx, the exploitation of one class of people by another is a crucial characteristic of capitalist economic systems. Entrepreneurs extract a "surplus value" in profit, which is the excess between the price of a product and the wage of workers producing the product. To the extent that capitalists extract surplus value from work they do not directly perform, they exploit the working class (Marx, 1906: v.1, pp. 708–709). Exploitation of the working class formed the primary injustice of the capitalist system which Marx criticized.

As we will discuss later, the sick may be broadly construed as a class of people, subject to financial exploitation under capitalism and bearing numerous similarities to the working class depicted in Marx's theoretical analysis. In this context it is not surprising that exploitation of the sick for profit would be viewed as reprehensible in socialist societies. These countries have either eliminated or strictly controlled the proliferation of competing pharmaceutical companies, insurance corporations, health equipment industries, proprietary hospitals, and nursing homes all of which extract profit from illness under capitalism. In most cases hospitals, ancillary facilities caring for the sick, and industries manufacturing health products are either owned or controlled by the state. Under these circumstances, profiteering through exploitation of illness is greatly reduced.

Contrasting value assumptions   Because it is so intimately related to the medicocivil structure, the organization of health services within a society depends to a great extent on its broad sociopolitical context. Similarly, the potential for change *within* the institution of medicine cannot be separated from broad sociopolitical change in a society. It is doubtful that a country can modify its medical care system substantially without more general sociopolitical re-organization like those which have accompanied the advent of socialist governmental systems in many countries.

Moreover, the potential for change reflects not only the concrete social structural arrangements of a given time and place, but also a society's basic values. For example, inhibitions against socialized medical services in the United States have origins deeper than the investments of capitalist enterprises in the health field. A society which highly values individualism, property rights, freedom of mobility, and personal as opposed to collective achievement cannot easily accept many of the limitations which socialism imposes. On the one hand, physicians trained under a capitalist system tend to protect jealously their right to practice autonomously, free from the controls of a federal administrative structure (Sade, 1971; Chapman and Talmadge, 1971). On the other hand, patients sometimes oppose the creation of a national health service because it would tend to restrict their freedom of choice in selecting a doctor.

It should be noted, however, that these objections to socialized medicine are essentially the objections of the upper middle class. Low-income patients possess little freedom of choice in their selection of physicians; they generally attend hospital outpatient clinics, where staff members care for them on a rotating basis with frequent turnover (Kosa et al., 1969). The values fostering private practice and fee-for-service health care do not necessarily support a system satisfactory to all citizens. In certain countries which have successfully improved the distribution of health services (for example, the People's Republic of China), individualistic values traditionally have held less prominence than collectivist values, or have been intentionally subordinated to collectivist values since the advent of socialism (Horn, 1969; cf. Hardin, 1968, 1972). One might propose that in the United States the very values that uphold individualism, property rights, free mobility, and personal achievement impede re-organizational measures which, though limiting the freedom of individual physicians, would ameliorate the severe distributional inequalities of American medicine.

Thus, to return to our initial question in this chapter, it is by no means clear that a humane health care system is possible in a capitalist society. The institution of medicine is intimately tied to the broad sociopolitical framework of a society. Under capitalism, the right of individual citizens to decent health care remains an ambiguous principle. Despite widespread concern about the costliness, maldistribution, and poor quality of services, the medical profession and large American corporations continue to exploit illness for profit. In this sociopolitical context, it is probably naive to presume that a responsive and effective health system can emerge through incremental reforms—without basic (and perhaps revolutionary) transformation of the social order.

Subsequently we will return to these problems. At this point, however, it is appropriate to consider several previous theoretical analyses of medicine as a social institution. In this brief review of theory in medical sociology, we are concerned primarily with those aspects of health and illness which contribute to the stability or change of larger social institutions or systems.

2   Social Theory and Medicine

Few social scientists have studied medical problems from the perspective of general social theory. Although numerous empirical studies have emerged, this work usually has not extended general theory; nor have broader theoretical frameworks shaped the direction of empirical research (cf. Merton, 1968:139–171). The rudimentary state of social theory in the health field has led to negative consequences on two levels. First, it has cast a pall on academic medical sociology, which has been viewed as an unexciting area by sociologists interested in broad theoretical issues. Secondly, medical sociology has proved largely irrelevant for most health workers and consumers. Though deeply concerned with social and psychological dimensions of patient care, activists despair to find a coherent theory which would aid them in their daily struggles toward a humane health system.

Three sociologists—Talcott Parsons, Eliot Freidson, and David Mechanic—have explained medical phenomena within a broader theoretical framework. Although all three have made significant contributions, their conclusions remain incomplete on the theoretical level and seldom have been helpful for workers concerned with ongoing problems of health care. Rather than attempting an exhaustive exposition and critique, our purpose here is to summarize some of the strengths and weaknesses of each theoretical position. Later we will incorporate elements of these analyses into an alternative theoretical framework, developed largely from socialist ideas.

PARSONS

The sick role   Parsons presented his classic analysis of medical practice as part of a general theoretical treatise on the nature of social systems (1951:428–479). For Parsons, illness must be viewed not strictly as a pathophysiological process but also as an inherently social phenom-enon. When people become ill, according to Parsons, they adopt a social role, characterized by four fairly standard role-expectations: (1) sick persons are not held "responsible" for their incapacity; (2) they are ex-empted from their usual role and task obligations; (3) they must want to leave the role and "get well" (that is, the legitimation of the sick role is conditional); (4) they are obliged to seek and comply with technically competent medical advice.

Parsons' achievement derives less from his exposition of these four role-expectations—which have been cogently criticized as highly variable in reality (Gordon, 1966)—than from the broader theoretical framework within which he places the sick role. *Illness,* in Parsons' analysis, *is one form of deviance* and consequently must be viewed *as a problem of social control.*

The roles which individuals must occupy in modern society often sub-ject them to great strains and pressures. Parsons devotes primary atten-tion to strains which arise in the occupational system and the nuclear family, but similar conflicts arise in a variety of other institutional settings (Parsons and Fox, 1952). The personal troubles which result from the roles society imposes can lead to dissatisfaction and frustration. Although Parsons never states it explicitly, the logical consequence of these strains is revolutionary action, in which individuals would unite to overthrow existing social systems with their oppressive role structures.

In his discussion of social control, Parsons hints at the revolutionary potential which the sick role helps to limit and contain:

> The criminal, being extruded from the company of 'decent' citizens, can only by coercion be prevented from joining up with his fellow criminals. . . . The conditional legitimation of the sick person's status on the other hand, places him in a special relation to people who are not sick, to the members of his family and to the various people in the health services, particularly physicians. This control is part of the price he pays for his partial legitimation, and it is clear that the basic structure resulting is that of the dependence of each sick person on a group of non-sick per-sons rather than of sick persons on each other. This in itself is highly important from the point of view of the social system since it **prevents the relevant motivations from spreading through either group formation or positive legitimation.** It is especially important that the motivational components, which cannot be expressed in the deviant behavior itself, in this case tend to tie the sick person to non-deviant people, rather than to other deviants, unlike the delinquent gang as analyzed above.
>
> But again, the sick role not only isolates and insulates, it also exposes the deviant to reintegrative forces (1951:312–313, emphasis added).

The sick role thus becomes a convenient tool to maintain the status quo. For individuals who encounter oppressive qualities of the social roles (familial, occupational, etc.) which are part of the objective conditions under which they must live, the sick role permits temporary deviance from usual role-expectations. It also isolates the deviant and prevents the group formation (such as the organization of dissident individuals) which would be needed for fundamental social change. In this sense, the sick role cools out the opposition.

Parsons has perceived the horror but remains unruffled. He correctly recognizes illness as one of several deviant routes which individuals may take in response to the strains they encounter in their social roles. The sick role is a particularly opportune mechanism of social control, however, since it permits limited deviance without threatening the social system's stability. There are two possible responses to this insight: satisfaction about society's methods of "reintegrating" troubled individuals under strain, or disappointment that the sick role may effectively stifle the dynamic conflict which is a source of basic change in society. Perhaps reflecting the conservative values for which he frequently has been criticized, Parsons seems to adopt the former response.

Social control of the sick: certification In Parsons' framework, doctors logically become agents of social control. They are the gatekeepers who regulate access to the sick role. People in trouble come to physicians; the latter enter into a process of investigation and negotiation by which they determine whether their clients may enter the sick role, temporarily leaving their customary roles at work, in the family, and so forth.

Essentially, physicians are responsible for "certifying" illness. Depending on the institutional context in which doctors and patients interact, certification may be formal or informal, and the criteria for certification may be strict or loose. In the setting of the nuclear family, for example, the private practitioner's verbal declaration that a client is sick suffices for exempting the patient from most familial role-expectations. In industry, the armed forces, and the military draft, on the other hand, the physician must provide written certification, which must be re-evaluated periodically, based on the patient's current status. Certification in all these latter settings usually is determined according to bureaucratically standardized criteria and is often difficult to obtain. (The institutional variability in certification is discussed in greater detail in Section 3).

In its social control function, the physician's role differs mainly in degree from analogous roles like policeman, judge, and clergyman. The policeman and judge act as certifiers of criminal deviance, the clergyman of moral or religious deviance. Often, particularly in the field of mental health, the medical role overlaps with the legal or religious role. Thus, a psychiatrist's decision can lead to incarceration in mental hospitals rather than prisons when clients are thought to be criminally insane (Szasz, 1963, 1972). As Parsons points out, in rendering judgments about acceptable or inappropriate behavior, the psychiatrist has taken on activities previously in the sphere of the minister of religion (Parsons, 1970:292–324; cf. Szasz, 1970).

Although Parsons recognizes these social control functions of the physician's role, his analysis is again uncritical. In regulating access to the sick role, the physician permits limited deviance for individuals who experience strain in their customary roles. From Parsons' perspective, this certification procedure has positive effects in limiting deviance and preserving social stability. However, Parsons does not consider in depth the actual strains which lead patients to seek certification in the first place. In certifying illness, doctors often deflect attention from the basic injustices and material grievances which trouble their patients in everyday life. Periodic entrance into the sick role helps people cope with their objective reality but also often defuses the anger and bitterness which leads to political organization and activism. Consequently, Parsons emphasizes individual adjustment within the sick role, causing adaptation rather than change in the social system.

The doctor-patient relationship   Because the physician acts as an agent of social control, his allegiance with the patient is often conditional and usually ambiguous. Parsons does not fully recognize the tension between the social control aspects of the doctor's role and the expectation of trust and confidence between physician and patient.

In his later writings on the doctor-patient relationship, Parsons describes the relationship as a collectivity. The patient, in this analysis, is not a passive object of therapy but an active participant, working closely with the physician toward the common goal of therapy:

> The classic "doctor-patient relationship" should then be considered to be the minimal relevant collectivity. It is the solidarity of this collectivity which constitutes the basis of mutual "trust" between physician and patient. . . . Looked at from this point of view, the contribution of the patient becomes immediately meaningful. . . . he is not, for instance, just a "consumer" but to some degree a "producer" of health service (1970:338).

This view of the doctor-patient relationship, though attractive and perhaps accurate in some settings, conflicts with the view of the physician as an agent of social control, regulating access to a deviant role. The former analysis depicts doctor and patient as close and trusting comrades, working in the best interests of the patient; in the latter viewpoint, the physician must make a detached and somewhat aloof judgment whether the patient's symptoms and signs qualify for certification of illness.

On balance, Parsons' analysis of the doctor-patient relationship leans in the direction of formality and distance between doctor and patient, rather than toward closeness and trust. For example, in his application of the pattern-variables to the role of the physician. Parsons describes in detail those features which create distance rather than closeness between doctor and patient (1951:55 ff., 433 ff.). In terms of the physician's scope of interest in the patient, the doctor-patient relationship is *functionally specific,* rather than diffuse. Therefore, in Parsons' analysis, the physician generally limits concern to the patient's health (and perhaps those other areas of the patient's life which directly affect health) and is less interested in matters which are not health-related. The doctor's emotional involvement in the relationship, according to Parsons, is also limited by the pattern of *affective-neutrality,* rather than affectivity. As Fox has pointed out, the physician's emotional involvement often becomes stronger than is implied by Parsons' original formulation—and is better characterized as "detached concern" than as "affective neutrality" (Fox, 1957). Nevertheless, even from this modified viewpoint, strong normative standards constrain the emotional ties between doctor and patient from becoming too intense.

Similarly, in Parsons' analysis the orientation of the physician is *universalistic* rather than particularistic. Thus the doctor does not react professionally to particular attributes of individual patients (physical attractiveness, financial status, educational background, etc.) which might create positive or negative feelings. Instead, while attending to the needs of individual patients, the doctor is expected to respond to those pathophysiological characteristics that make any patient similar to other patients with the same disease. According to Parsons, the doctor-patient relationship emphasizes *achievement,* not ascriptive qualities. Physician and patient focus their expectations on the doctor's performance of skills and success in achieving therapeutic results. In this framework, attention is directed away from those ascriptive traits (such as sex, race, ethnic background, etc.) which would tend to draw the doctor and patient together or pull them apart on a personal level. Considering the physician's private interests, Parsons depicts the normative pattern as *collectivity-orientation,* rather than self-orientation. In contrast to the businessman, the profession of medicine emphasizes the doctor's obligation to place the patient's welfare above one's personal interests, particularly economic interests. As a result, according to Parsons, strong sanctions have arisen which restrict commercialism and the profit motive in medicine.

Parsons intends his application of the pattern-variables as a statement of the broad normative principles which govern professional behavior. He does not present his formulation as an accurate account of the actual behavior of doctors and patients. In various medical practices, a greater or lesser discrepancy may exist between the normative pattern and empirical reality. For example, in recent years physicians' behavior—especially in reaction to increased government spending for health care—has shown obvious economic self-interest and dubious collectivity-orientation (Lewis and Keairnes, 1970; Freidson, 1970a).

More importantly, the normative patterns Parsons describes reinforce the social control elements of the doctor's role and limit the unconditional allegiance with patients. Functional specificity implies that the doctor should not have broader contact with patients outside the medical sphere; this would prevent doctors and patients from working together toward common political goals. Affective neutrality and universalism mean that the emotional bonds of friendship and the particular personal characteristics which might unite doctors and patients in non-medical activities are discouraged. Achievement orientation focuses attention on the success or failure of concrete therapeutic maneuvers, rather than on the strength of the ongoing relationship between doctor and patient. Collectivity-orientation is the only normative pattern Parsons describes which brings doctors closer to patients rather than more distant from them.

It might be argued, as Parsons implies, that the distancing mechanisms invoked by these normative patterns are necessary in a professional relationship, where the intimacy involved in history-taking and the physical examination might create conflicts. In addition, the psychic problems of handling dying and death would be more severe for physicians who shared affective, ascriptive, diffuse, and particularistic ties with their patients. On the other hand, these same normative patterns allow physicians to act more effectively as agents of social control, relatively detached from their patients' objective living conditions and emotional concerns. To the extent that doctors' allegiance with their patients is not unconditional, they may at times serve the interests of the social order more than those of the people they claim to help. The normative patterns which detach doctors from their patients' suffering encourage physicians to act as gatekeepers in certifying the sick role. These same patterns inhibit doctors from allying with their patients in fighting the sociopolitical conditions which often are the source of suffering and the impetus to seek certification as ill.

The competence gap: a source of social stratification in medicine
Technical knowledge is differentially distributed in society. Professional education involves the acquisition of facts, skills, and methodologies which laymen do not share. The differential possession of technical knowledge is one source of professionals' power to shape the actions of their clients. In this sense the "competence gap" between professionals and clients creates a stratified relationship, in which professionals hold a superordinate position and clients occupy a subordinate one.

Parsons describes the competence gap, and the resulting stratification of professional-client relationships, as follows:

> Relative to its relevant "laity," the professional relation is by its nature asymmetrical and thereby drastically different from the democratic associational relationship among "peers." In one essential aspect, the primary axis of this asymmetry lies in the superior competence of the professional. . . . Seeking the services of a competent physician or lawyer is different from peers "agreeing" about what should be done in a distressing situation. . . . In all . . . these basic respects, there exists a "competence gap" between professionals and lay persons (1969:336).

Ignorance of the somatic processes of illness and the physiologic basis of therapy, of course, is one of the most frightening aspects of being a patient. When people come to a doctor, they in some sense surrender control over the body to another individual, who presumably understands the maneuvers necessary for healing. The physician's superordinate status, as compared to the patient's relative helplessness, raises the potential problem of exploitation; because of the competence gap, doctors are in a position to take advantage of patients' technical ignorance.

According to Parsons, this stratification must be mollified by the emotional ties between doctor and patient. He describes these ties under the rubric of "trust":

> If the necessary lay cooperation with the professional is to be assured, it cannot rest on the layman's full understanding of "what the professional is doing" in a sense presupposed by the slogan **caveat emptor** in the market field. There must be bases of trusted validation of competence other than the typical layman's personal competence to evaluate it. . . . Such a competence gap must be bridged by something like what we call trust (1969:336).

If sufficient trust exists, Parsons implies, stratification poses no great problem; doctors and patients may unite in a trusting collectivity working toward the common goal of therapy.

As occurs frequently in his analyses of the professions, Parsons paints too sanguine a picture. Is the competence gap (and the stratification it implies) a *necessary* feature of professional-client relationships, or is it simply a description of professional dominance? Empirically (as we discuss in Section 4) physicians tend to withhold information about illness and therapy in a wide variety of circumstances. The most obvious instance of information withholding centers on hesitancy to communicate the diagnosis of fatal illness. However, doctors often do not provide explanations to patients with non-fatal and even trivial problems. In fact, numerous studies have shown that patients in the United States and Britain are more dissatisfied about doctors' reluctance to provide sufficient information than about any other aspect of medical care.

There appears to be little reason for this low level of communication, other than the preservation of physicians' dominant position in the doctor-patient relationship. To the extent that doctors try to narrow the competence gap by offering detailed explanations of illness and therapy, they also give up the power which depends on patients' ignorance. Norms which foster information withholding maintain the stratified nature of the doctor-patient relationship. In this sense the competence gap is not a necessary feature of professional-client relationships. Instead, it is a structural factor which prevents doctors from interacting as equals with fully informed patients. By reinforcing professional dominance, the competence gap also inhibits doctors and patients from uniting to combat those social conditions which often motivate patients to enter the sick role.

Social control of physicians: professionalism Because of patients' relative helplessness, they occupy a vulnerable position. Physicians have power over patients which derives from an asymmetry of technical knowledge and skills. As discussed previously, doctors also often act as agents of social control, regulating access to the sick role. In brief, patients are a potentially exploitable group in society. What restrains doctors from taking advantage (particularly financially but also in other ways) of their patients?

According to Parsons, physicians are subject to broad standards to which he variously refers as "professionalism," or "the professional complex." Parsons sees the social control of physicians as deriving not from external agencies which monitor the behavior of individual practitioners, but rather from the profession itself:

> To use the medical case for reference, the principle of **caveat emptor** for the purchaser of health services will scarcely be adequate as a basis for accountability. Nor will legal liability be sufficient, if this must be enforced by judges and attorneys who are not technically competent at professional levels in anything but the law; and if the initiative is left to litigants who conceive themselves to be injured and are willing and financially able to assume the burden of litigation. Nor can accountability reside with administrators who are not themselves professionally competent in the subject matter in question, nor with grievance procedures, nor, finally, with the "decent opinion of mankind" as expressed through the mass communication system. Professional groups must, to some essential degree, be self-regulating, taking responsibility for the technical standards of their integrity in serving societal functions (1969:330).

Presumably, professional norms prevent the exploitation of patients and mitigate the dangers of the competence gap. The primary normative pattern which limits potential exploitation in Parsons' analysis is collectivity-orientation (1951:463–464). Because it curtails advertising, bargaining over fees, and other self-interested economic behaviors which are common in the business world, this normative pattern encourages physicians to concern themselves with their patients' welfare above considerations of personal profit.

Again, Parsons' notion of a self-regulating medical profession is over-optimistic. Empirically, American physicians have not exhibited notable economic self-restraint, despite the normative patterns Parsons describes. Individual practitioners have been free to determine the conditions of their practice, relatively independently from governmental or consumer control. This situation has resulted in severe maldistribution of personnel, high fees (often increasing exorbitantly in response to increased government health expenditures), and poor quality when assessed by objective standards (e.g., Peterson et al., 1956; Lewis and Hassanein, 1970).

In fact, numerous critics are now asserting that professional dominance is one of the primary problems facing American medicine today. From this latter viewpoint, the freedom of individual practitioners must be brought under the tighter scrutiny of monitoring groups based outside the profession. The growing opinion is that professional self-regulation has not functioned effectively in medicine, and that the social control of doctors' behavior must move away from the professional standards set by doctors themselves.

In summary, Parsons' contributions to the field of medical sociology have been extremely important because they have always been tied to a more general theoretical framework. Parsons has elucidated the sick role as a deviant role in society. In this context, physicians may act as agents of social control. They serve to maintain the existing social order by certifying illness, thus providing a temporary exemption for individuals who encounter strain in their usual roles. The doctor-patient relationship, in Parsons' view, tends to be a formal and distant relationship, in which the competence gap creates an inherent source of stratification. The principal problems in Parsons' analysis center on an uncritical acceptance of physicians' social control functions, his inattention to the ways in which physicians' behavior may inhibit change in society, and an over-optimism about the medical profession's ability to regulate itself and to prevent the exploitation of individual patients.

FREIDSON

The problem of professionalism Parsons' kindness to the profession of medicine provides a suitable foil for Freidson's jaundiced eye. Freidson has formulated a wide-ranging critique of the medical profession and has observed medical phenomena within a broader theory of professions in general. Rather than reviewing Freidson's significant contributions, it is worthwhile to focus on several of his conclusions and to consider their more problematic aspects.

For Freidson, the profession's autonomy to control the conditions of day-to-day professional activities poses the central threat to specific clients and to the public at large. Unlike Parsons, Freidson does not trust the profession's capacity to regulate itself through broad normative patterns. He criticizes Parsons' acceptance of the public stance of the profession; he doubts that a continuity exists between the normative patterns Parsons describes and the empirical behavior of practicing physicians. Although collectivity-orientation is the profession's normative stance, Freidson claims, it cannot be assumed that doctors' concrete behavior reflects these norms. Therefore, normative expectations must be distinguished from actual performance:

> The "collectivity or service orientation" usually refers to the orientation of **individual** members of an occupation rather than to organizations. But clearly, the attitudes of individuals constitute an entirely different kind of criterion than the attributes of occupational institutions. . . . But curiously enough, there appears to be no reliable information which actually demonstrates that a service orientation is in fact strong and widespread among professionals. . . .
>
> Parsons does not specify performance at all, but only expectation. Furthermore, those expectations are part of the broad institutional norms connected with professions as officially organized occupations. They are, in fact, the normative segment of the formal organization of professions, expressed by codes of ethics, public statements of spokesmen for the profession, and the like. They are quite distinct, analytically and empirically, from the actual norms of individual professionals. . . . More

concrete norms seem necessary for the analysis of medical work (Freidson, 1970a:80–81, 160).

From this viewpoint, the service or (in Parsons' terms) collectivity-orientation of the medical profession does not necessarily describe the orientation of individual practitioners, but rather reflects the publicly propounded norms of the profession. As Freidson points out, it is difficult to reconcile collectivity-orientation with the present crisis in American medical care—a crisis caused largely by doctors' often exorbitant fees and their disinclination to practice in areas of the country where many low-income patients reside.

Because he doubts the profession's ability to regulate itself, Freidson discounts the importance of practitioners' autonomy in controlling the conditions of practice. According to Freidson, members of all occupations seek this autonomy, but only the professions justify autonomy on the basis of special expertise. The medical profession claims that doctors' elaborate training and technical knowledge imply that only other doctors can determine who is qualified to practice medicine and what kinds of practice are appropriate. In fact, Freidson claims, the profession exerts very minimal control over the quality of medical care (1970b:101). The possession of technical knowledge, in this view, does not in itself justify professional autonomy; the "knowledge of *how to apply"* technical knowledge most effectively is not necessarily part of the competence of doctors as opposed to that of administrators, patients, or politicians (Freidson, 1970a:344).

The profession's quest for autonomy resembles that of other occupations but has a more sophisticated ideological line. Because the profession has failed to institute effective review procedures, Freidson claims, individual practitioners have been free to charge "all that the helpless traffic will bear rather than only the decent income to which the practitioner is entitled" (1970a:363). Freidson continues:

> *Given such a failure, there seems to be little justification to the profession's claim of autonomy over the economic terms of work. . . . In setting both the economic and the social terms of work, the material interests of the profession should of course be recognized, represented, and at least partially satisfied, but such interests are little more "professional" than are those of trade unions. Indeed, so far as the terms of work go, professions differ from trade unions only in their sanctimoniousness (1970a: 364–365,367).*

In Freidson's opinion, technical training and the life-and-death nature of many medical activities are not sufficient reason for professional autonomy. To quote the paraphrase of Clemenceau, medicine is too important to be left to the doctors.

Freidson also makes explicit the problem of stratification within the doctor-patient relationship. As discussed previously, Parsons minimizes this stratification by claiming that the competence gap is bridged by trust. Expertise and possession of specialized knowledge place the physician, almost inevitably, in a superordinate position. Professional dominance, according to Freidson, can be overcome only with great difficulty in organized medical settings such as hospitals. Furthermore, the competence gap implies inequality within the doctor-patient relationship. That is, despite norms requiring patients' "informed consent" to diagnostic and therapeutic procedures, and despite an increasing consumer participation in health policy, stratification remains inherent because of the differential possession of technical knowledge:

> And this points to the most profound problem of utopian equalitarianism —how individuality and equal participation in communal decisions can be maintained in the face of special competencies. . . . So long as the goal of therapy is maintained and physicians are held to know how to achieve it, physicians will maintain a place of privilege and "authority" . . . (Freidson, 1970b:175–176).

Through specialized competence, the professional holds power over the client. By seeking help, always in relative ignorance, the client necessarily assumes a subordinate position.

One way the professional preserves the privileged position vis-a-vis the client is through the manipulation of information. Perhaps to a greater extent than other professionals, as previously mentioned, physicians maintain power within the doctor-patient relationship by withholding pertinent information about diagnosis and therapy. According to Freidson, when doctors give information, they provide a basis upon which patients can independently decide whether to accept or reject physicians' recommendations; this creates "management problems." To the extent that advice and decisions must be explained and justified to a layman, the doctor's privileged position is jeopardized. As a result, physicians tend to encourage patients' "faith" or "trust," rather than relying on processes of persuasion. Freidson concludes: "Insistence on faith constitutes insistence that the client give up his role as an independent adult and, by so neutralizing him, protect the esoteric foundation of the profession's institutionalized authority" (1970b:143).

In short, while Parsons is confident about the profession's capacity for self-regulation and about trust as a mechanism to mollify the competence gap, Freidson is much less sanguine. For Freidson, professional autonomy and dominance have become crucial problems in the current crisis of health care. The picture Freidson paints is bleak. What solutions does he offer?

Control of professional autonomy: political implications The implications of Freidson's analysis for change are rather limited and, to the extent he states them explicitly, depressing. There is a sense of inevitability in Freidson's work which is unwarranted, both theoretically and in terms of present empirical reality. Where differential distribution of technical knowledge exists, Freidson implies, professional dominance emerges. Freidson sets up the beginnings of a dialectic, by which inequality of technical training produces a tendency toward stratification in professional-client relationships. Conflict and change are logical outcomes of professsional dominance, part of the dialectic Freidson introduces but does not completely formulate. The consumer movement and the drive toward community control over local health services are empirical manifestations of conflict which derive largely from patients' growing dissatisfaction with professional dominance. Freidson is correct in specifying and criticizing the stratification which is inherent in the differential distribution of knowledge among doctors and patients. But he does not go far enough in describing the dynamic tensions of this stratification, the potential for conflict, and the possibilities for change.

The modifications in policy which Freidson suggests are quite modest and, if implemented, would not lead to major innovations in the health care system. Most notably, Freidson believes that private practice, based on fee for service, should be continued. The fee-for-service system, he claims, allows the patient freedom to choose from available practitioners:

*Only a system that provides the individual patient himself with the opportunities and resources to exercise his own choice of practitioner and service is likely to sustain such human standards. In evaluating that problem in the light of paying the physician, it seems to me that the most flexible and direct method of supplying individual patients with such choice as individuals (rather than as members of some organized group negotiating contracts) is the fee-for-service method. By the nature of the method, one patient's decision to use a physician's services is directly and immediately translated into a financial benefit to the practitioner chosen. This does not mean that a capitation or salary basis of payment cannot be set up in a way that allows fairly flexible patient choice, but only that fee-for-service provides the most direct and **immediately consequential** means for doing so (1970b:218–219, emphasis in original).*

According to Freidson, low-income patients should receive assistance from some type of insurance, perhaps national in scope. Moreover, the fee and insurance structures as a whole should be more carefully monitored by a formal administrative apparatus (1970b:216-225). In Freidson's proposals for reform, however, private fee-for-service practice would continue to occupy a central position in a pluralist health system.

The economics of this argument are naive. Low-income patients in the United States have never had the freedom to choose practitioners since their very ability to pay has been limited. Such patients most often have resorted to hospital outpatient departments and emergency rooms, where they could exert no choice over the rotating house staff who have cared for their needs. Even if a national health insurance system is established that would enable low-income patients to pay private doctors' fees (as discussed in Section 5), it would not correct the maldistribution of personnel and facilities which prevents patients in rural and many urban areas from receiving adequate medical care. Freidson's optimism about private practice based on fee-for-service, given its dismal record, is surprising.

Furthermore, the controls over professional dominance and autonomy which Freidson proposes would not lead to fundamental shifts in the present medical power structure. Freidson believes that the autonomy of professionals must be limited by carefully devised administrative structures. The precise nature and composition of these structures, however, remain unclear from Freidson's analysis. Freidson seems to indicate that control of professional autonomy would emerge from formal review mechanisms, rather than the largely informal procedures which now are prevalent in medical circles. Formal periodic internal review (that is, review by medical professionals) would be combined with formal periodic outside review by other professionals who are not themselves physicians (1970b: 222-225). Although Freidson never explicates who these "outside" professionals might be, one assumes they would be medical sociologists, basic scientists, lawyers, and other highly trained individuals. Presumably these people would be capable of evaluating professional performance according to some unspecified objective criteria.

Although Freidson's proposals for improving the health care system aim toward formal review procedures, they would not create basic changes in control over health policy. "Outside" professional review would merely shift the locus of power, away from physicians as the sole review body and toward a mixed review agency, also composed of professionals. The elite nature of professional governance would remain intact. In view of the actual decision-making processes of many hospitals, which are formally controlled by non-medical boards composed largely of other professionals, the true power over policy decisions probably would continue to rest with the doctors.

Freidson does offer the consumer a role in policy making, but again this role would be ponderous and formal. Although he claims that there is "no substitute" for the direct expression of "interests and needs by the patient himself," Freidson proposes that consumers state their preferences through a "formal vote of confidence" in health services (1970b: 225-231). Despite this parliamentary imagery, it is unclear how a vote of no confidence would make any difference if medical care continues to be organized along the lines of private, fee-for-service practice. What effect would it have, after all, if the people of Appalachia or urban low-income areas expressed lack of confidence in their physicians, when in fact they cannot even gain access to physicians? Democratic procedures will not change doctors' autonomy to practice where and how they wish.

On the other hand, Freidson opposes substantive control over health services by organized consumers. He is extremely skeptical about the potentialities of community control and feels that interest in community participation will decline in the future:

> It will decline because of the institutionalization attending reform, because of the professionalization of the community participants, because of the attrition of enthusiasm by the tedious pace of peaceful change, because of the rise of other issues to attention, and because of the irreducible fact that expertise does exist and is needed for the public good

in so many areas as to make it virtually impossible to explain and debate
every one (1970a:381).

In this way the control mechanisms Freidson suggests remain weak at both the national and local levels. Nationally, since Freidson believes private, fee-for-service practice should be maintained, controls would be exerted only by formal review bodies composed of medical and non-medical professionals. There would certainly be no socialized organization, by which physicians would be required to work for the government and within which professional performance would be reviewed by organized consumers. Locally, in Freidson's view, patients could express their feelings through formal votes of confidence or no confidence. But according to Freidson, local governing bodies, in which consumers would control the medical personnel and organization of services within their own communities, would prove ineffective.

In addition to the modest control mechanisms he proposes, Freidson's analysis suffers from a lack of broader sociopolitical analysis; he accepts as given the present sociopolitical system of the United States. Any change in health policy limiting professional autonomy would occur within a system similar to the present one. Freidson offers his recommendations for change under the rubric of a section heading entitled, "Consulting Professions in a Free Society" (1970a:333). It is interesting to note that Freidson never defines precisely what he means by the term, "free society." Presumably it is a society which resembles current American society but exerts tighter constraints on professional autonomy. But, as often has been asked, is a society free when significant stratification exists? Is it free when it experiences severe maldistribution of goods and services?

Freidson realizes that necessary improvements in medical care will emerge only when doctors are less "free" to practice as they wish. But he does not adequately extend his analysis to consider the broader sociopolitical changes which are the necessary concomitants of adequate controls over professional autonomy. The record shows (as will be discussed in greater detail in Section 6) that the controls needed to improve the distribution of medical services emerge only when governments move in the direction of socialism. While Freidson's critique of professionalism is trenchant, the various reformist proposals he suggests will not succeed without broader sociopolitical change in the United States. As a social institution, medicine is intimately tied to the economic, political, and other subsystems of the society. Modified controls of professional behavior within medicine cannot occur independently of alterations in these other subsystems as well. In fact, it might be argued that change within medicine must be predicated on change in the society at large.

Illness as deviance versus illness as suffering Although Freidson analyzes professional autonomy and professional dominance as two major problems in American society, his tone is remarkably detached, dispassionate, and apolitical. In a sense, Freidson adopts as a goal the mild-mannered stance of the observer, which he feels will be more helpful ultimately than a too-close involvement in the immediate problems of clinical practice. He states:

> *Collaborating with medicine in its institutionalized tasks requires adopt-*
> *ing that distorted view with all its deficiencies. Studying it as an*
> *outsider allows one to see medicine as one of a number of human institu-*
> *tions, reflecting one of many intellectual points of view, one of many*
> *moral standpoints, and expressing the material and ideological com-*
> *mitments of only one of many organized groups in our society (1970b:42).*

Freidson gives himself credit for his ability to stand back from the medical profession and believes that the sharpness of his critique depends, at least in part, on his own distance from the ongoing tensions and pressures of clinical work. He properly refers to himself, using a classfication developed earlier by Robert Straus, as writing a "sociology *of* medicine," rather than practicing "sociology *in* medicine" (Strauss, 1957).

But distance has its drawbacks too. Although Freidson incisively criticizes the profession, he does not adequately convey the pain and suffering with which professionals must deal. It can be argued that some of the behavioral patterns which Freidson describes under the rubric of "professional dominance" represent adaptive mechanisms, which aid human beings who make life-and-death decisions in the face of suffering. Especially in critical situations, the physician's assumption of a superordinate role in decision-making is perhaps the only appropriate response. Of course, this does not dilute the impact of Freidson's argument that, especially in less critical situations, professional dominance and autonomy do not serve the public interest.

More important than his distance from doctors' experience of suffering, however, is Freidson's detachment from the suffering of patients themselves. Freidson bases his analysis of illness on the concept of deviance. He claims that all illness represents social deviance and elaborates Parsons' original exposition of this idea. Comparing illness and crime, Freidson proposes that, in general, crimes are deviant acts for which an individual is held responsible, while illnesses comprise deviant states for which an individual is not held responsible. Freidson develops a typology of illness as deviance by which the deviance is viewed as minor or serious, and as illegitimate, conditionally legitimate, or unconditionally legitimate. Thus, for example, a "cold" would be considered a minor, conditionally legitimate form of deviance involving a temporary suspension of a few ordinary obligations, a temporary enhancement of ordinary privileges, and an obligation to get well. On the other hand, cancer is a serious, unconditionally legitimate deviance, marked by a permanent suspension of many ordinary obligations and a marked addition to privileges (1970a:239).

While Freidson's typology is a useful theoretical advance over Parsons' formulation, it manifests a curious degree of disinterest. Freidson never seems to involve himself emotionally in the suffering of the patients he classifies. Cancer, after all, is not only a serious, unconditionally legitimate deviance; it is also a painful, emotionally devastating experience. The experiential quality of illness eludes Freidson's theoretical exposition. In addition, the helpless position of the sick—which is the source of their potential exploitation by physicians, hospitals, the insurance and pharmaceutical industries, etc.—is not conveyed sensitively in Freidson's writing. Finally, Freidson minimizes the conflicts between personality needs and the demands of the patient's social situation; as we discuss in Section 3, these conflicts often motivate individuals to deviate from their usual roles and to enter the sick role.

Although his detachment has aided Freidson in criticizing the profession, it has also prevented him from considering the central experiential and emotional qualities of being ill. Illness is indeed a form of social deviance, but it is more than that. It also involves suffering, conflict, helplessness, and potential exploitation. Just as Freidson's important work neglects the full political implications of bringing professional autonomy under tighter control, his theoretical analysis of illness as deviance minimizes the patient's experiential situation.

MECHANIC

Illness behavior   David Mechanic has contributed a variety of empirical studies to the literature of medical sociology; this work has focused on social psychological dimensions of medical care, comparative international analysis of health systems, and the problems of mental illness and social stress. His major theoretical advance has been the concept of "illness behavior," which he defines as follows:

> By this term we refer to the ways in which given symptoms may be differentially perceived, evaluated, and acted (or not acted) upon by different kinds of persons. Whether by reason of earlier experiences with illness, differential training in respect to symptoms, or whatever, some persons will make light of symptoms, shrug them off, avoid seeking medical care; others will respond to the slightest twinges of pain or discomfort by quickly seeking such medical care as is available. In short the realm of illness behavior falls logically and chronologically between two major traditional concerns of medical science: etiology and therapy. Variables affecting illness behavior come into play prior to medical scrutiny and treatment, but after etiological processes have been initiated. In this sense, illness behavior even determines whether diagnosis and treatment will begin at all (1962:189).

Illness behavior, then, comprises the different actions which individuals take in response to symptoms. The various backgrounds and experiences of individual patients pattern their illness behavior in predictable ways.

Mechanic has investigated the relationships between several characteristics of patients and their illness behavior. In operationalizing illness behavior, Mechanic has treated it as an essentially psychological dimension. He assesses the "tendency to adopt the sick role" (TASR) by constructing a score from students' answers to questionnaire items. For example:

> *During the past school year would you have reported to the University Health Services in the following hypothetical situations? A) You have been feeling poorly for a few days; B) You felt you had a temperature of about 100°; C) You felt you had a temperature of about 101°. [Answers: (0) certainly, (1) probably, (2) not very likely, (3) very unlikely] (Mechanic and Volkart, 1960:89; 1961:55).*

After operationalizing illness behavior in this way, Mechanic determines the statistical correlations between TASR and several other variables: patients' perceived stress, illness categories with which patients are diagnosed, and patients' religion (Mechanic and Volkart, 1960:90-94; Mechanic, 1962:190-192). He also finds that TASR, measured by questionnaire, significantly discriminates frequent from infrequent users of a university health service (Mechanic and Volkart, 1961:55-57). (The generalizability of these studies, done with middle class students, to the population at large is of course questionable.) Finally, in reviewing others' research, Mechanic discusses the influence of several other variables on illness behavior: social class, ethnic background, age, sex, educational experience, and perceptions of personal vulnerability (1962:190; 1968:236-270; 1972).

Each patient, after all, is unique. Mechanic helps us understand how a given patient's personal life experience shapes the reaction to symptoms. Some people suffer in silence; others are more voluble.

Predicting illness behavior: individual versus institutional characteristics
Yet Mechanic's analysis usually remains one-dimensional. He tends to ignore the basic question: *why* does patients' illness behavior vary in the ways he describes? For example, why do lower-income patients visit doctors less often? Why do people who perceive themselves under stress use medical facilities frequently? How do individuals develop the feelings of personal vulnerability which lead them to seek help? One leaves Mechanic's writings with a sense of determinism, as though the life history of the individual were the primary determinant of the patient's medical experience. Ultimately it is the variability among patients, rather than the similarity of their situation, which Mechanic emphasizes. On balance, what happens to a patient seems to depend on the kind of person he or she is, rather than the kind of medical institutions and personnel with whom a patient must deal.

Occasionally Mechanic tips his hat to the institutional constraints which affect patients' perceptions and reactions to their bodily processes. Like Freidson, Mechanic views illness as deviant behavior, though he adds little to Parsons' earlier formulation (Mechanic, 1968:15-48). Mechanic also discusses a number of institutional settings, such as the totalitarian state and the armed forces, in which the role demands that individuals experience are often severe, and where the sick role provides a convenient route for deviant behavior (1959). There are few references to institutional or social structural characteristics in Mechanic's work. Instead, he usually adopts a more typically clinical approach, studying the characteristics of patients rather than doctors, professional associations, or industries which capitalize on ill health.

However, there are good institutional reasons why different kinds of patients act as they do. For example, adopting an institutional perspective, one can provide fairly straightforward answers to the questions posed above about the variability of illness behavior. Lower-income patients do not utilize health facilities infrequently simply because they have little money (though, obviously, lack of money also deters them from visiting private practitioners who charge a standard fee for service). More than other groups in society, the poor must use hospital emergency rooms and outpatient departments, where they encounter impersonality, bureaucratization, and a rapid staff turnover. Although the availability of third-party welfare benefits for health care (Medicare, Medicaid, etc.) has modified this situation to a limited extent, the basic pattern persists (Kosa et al., 1969). Thus it is not only the individual characteristics of low-income people which determine the poor utilization of facilities; it is also the nature of the facilities to which they must turn.

Similarly, one can view the feelings of stress and personal vulnerability at two levels. Mechanic sees them essentially as the psychological traits of individuals. On the other hand, stress and vulnerability are not only matters of individual psychology. More often than not, these feelings emerge from painful qualities of the social structures within which individuals must function on a day-to-day basis. The "politics" (to cite Laing's usage) of family life, occupations, educational institutions, and leisure activities frequently are sources of great stress. Sensitive individuals are in fact vulnerable to this stress and react to it in several ways (Laing, 1969; 1972). Coping is the "normal" response. Other reactions are outright rebellion, which is rare, and illness behavior, which is common. In this sense, illness behavior (whether it involves emotional or physical symptomatology) represents an adaptive response to social structures which, to a greater or lesser degree, are oppressive.

Mechanic's analysis glosses the institutional factors involved in the genesis of illness behavior. It also overlooks the ways in which illness behavior, by permitting an easily controllable form of deviance, fosters institutional stability. When individuals adopt the sick role, the social problems from which their distress often derives remain unchallenged. Illness behavior, as an alternative to "coping" with social conditions which cause suffering, poses no threat to the status quo.

In fact, the question of stability and change represents a most significant hiatus in Mechanic's theoretical work. People who experience stress or who perceive themselves as especially vulnerable may show illness behavior. Mechanic emphasizes the behavioral manifestations of patients' suffering, rather than suffering's structural bases; he focuses on individual pain, not on social sickness. Yet in a society whose institutions often evoke illness behavior, social theory should move beyond descriptions of adjustment, to issues of change (Israel, 1971; Mills, 1967; Angel, 1971). From this perspective, illness behavior can be seen, at least in part, as a reflection of patients' stressful experience of the institutions with which they must deal. Often, it is also a conservative mechanism by which individuals can express pain without threatening social stability.

AN ALTERNATIVE THEORETICAL APPROACH

Because suffering has more than academic interest, social theory should be more than a matter of academic curiosity. As the major theoreticians of health and illness, Parsons, Freidson, and Mechanic uncover many seeds of despair in the vicissitudes of social structure. In doing so, however, they seldom lose their equanimity. As a result, their major advances seldom appear relevant to health workers and consumers. The latter are disgusted with the present health system and engage in scattered battles for change. In these struggles, they search for an informed theoretical framework, which would aid in their critique of current conditions and would point toward directions and tactics of change. The impatience of health workers and consumers with the literature of medical sociology is understandable.

In the sections that follow, we try to formulate a tentative theoretical framework which may be more useful for the health movement. The general orientation is that of Marxian analysis, although—as will become obvious—the analogies between the health system and the economic system of socialist theory are often somewhat tenuous. Nevertheless, the adoption of a Marxian framework permits a more detailed consideration of conflict within the health system. In addition, by analyzing the sources of stability and change, it clarifies some directions in which health workers and consumers may move in their day-to-day struggles.

Several themes recur in this theoretical framework: illness as a source of exploitation, the sick role as a conservative mechanism fostering social stability (Section 3), stratification in medicine (Section 4), and the imperialism of large medical institutions and health-related industries (Section 5). All these themes are extensions of classic socialist ideas. The aim is not to force all medical phenomena into a Marxian paradigm. Rather it is to use analogies from socialist theory in building an empirically relevant and politically meaningful analysis.

The sick role and social stability As frequently described, there are two major models of the desirable state for any social system. The first, an equilibrium model, analyzes social structure in terms of its functional consequences for preserving the status quo. From this point of view, deviance becomes a problem of social control, since it threatens to disrupt social stability. To a great extent Parsons' theory adopts this orientation: the sick role is functional because it allows temporary deviance from usual role expectations while maintaining social equilibrium.

In contrast, a dialectic model emphasizes the importance of social change. In a dialectic sense, conflict is viewed as a positive prerequisite to change in society. From this perspective the sick role may stabilize social structures which are oppressive for individuals or classes of individuals within society. A conflict analysis suggests that the sick role prevents individuals and groups from addressing the real sources of strain which may reside in social structure. Insofar as adoption of the sick role relieves strains which otherwise could become a focus of dissatisfaction and conflict, it becomes a conservative (and sometimes counterrevolutionary) mechanism inhibiting social change.

Stratification in medicine Also derived from Marxian theory is the notion of a stratified health system. In his analysis, Marx emphasizes differences among social classes based on their relation to the means of economic production. Economic roles and wages are only one of several criteria for stratification within society. Others include education, housing, and medical care; thus, different classes have differential access to health services.

Within the institution of medicine itself, Marx's notion of class may be applied to various groupings of health workers, administrators, and patients. Stratified according to their variable possession of medical authority, these groupings may have interests that conflict with one another. Like the worker who is subordinated to the capitalist within the economic structure, the patient is subordinated to health professionals and administrators in the medical hierarchy. The potential for exploitation of patients occurs in the health system, much as exploitation of workers is present in a capitalist economic system.

In addition, stratification occurs in the doctor-patient relationship itself, based on differential access to medical information. As we discuss later, doctors often preserve control over patients by withholding information about illness and therapy. This type of stratification, deriving from restricted communication, also creates the potential for conflict.

Medical imperialism Increasingly, American health care is taking on characteristics of big business. Financial strength and prestige are becoming concentrated in the hands of a few organizations participating in health care delivery. This trend toward monopoly parallels the growth of monopoly capital described by Lenin (1939) and others (e.g. Baran and Sweezy, 1966). The transition from a competitive capitalist market to domination by giant monopolies resembles changes which have occurred in the American health system. In medicine the locus of economic and political power has moved from entrepreneurship of individual physicians to corporate enterprise. This trend is reminiscent of monopolist combines in Lenin's analysis. In both cases resources are controlled by a few interlocking organizations. In Lenin's scheme the working class bears the burden of capitalist monopoly. By analogy we suggest that it is patients who suffer at the hands of a monolithic medical-industrial power structure.

The expansion of medical facilities and health-related industries is not unlike the imperialism of capitalist monopolies. Lenin notes the tendency for monopolist enterprises to expand into the international colonial sphere. Such expansion was legitimated in terms of a helping ideology whereby colonial development would be aided by imperialist corporations. Proponents of medical expansion also invoke a helping ideology to legitimate empire building—a process which actually maintains and enhances professional and corporate dominance of the health system, often at the expense of patients and other groups in society.

With the increasing commercialization of medical services, health care has been transformed into a commodity; as such, it is bought and sold like other goods and services. Because the demand for health care is virtually limitless, individual professionals and medical-industrial corporations have discovered great sources of profit in illness. Like the exploitation of workers by capitalists in Marx's scheme, the enterprises of medical capitalism do not hesitate to exploit patients. Medical imperialism contributes to this process, since patients ultimately bear the burden of medical expansion in the form of rising health costs. Because the power distribution in American medicine favors the providers rather than the consumers of health care, exploitation of illness and suffering persists.

Later, we discuss the themes of stratification and imperialism in greater detail. First, we consider the mechanisms by which the sick role contributes to social stability and inhibits change in society.

3   The Sick Role, Social Stability, and Social Change

Gus Tyler has said that any civilization gets the criminals it deserves. According to Tyler, crime is embedded in culture; tendencies toward lawlessness in the United States are supported by enduring cultural patterns (1962). Walter Lippmann (1962) and others have described "the underworld as a servant," performing those services which convention may condemn but human appetites crave. While laws formally maintain society's normative order, organized crime provides drugs, prostitutes, liquor, or gambling opportunities—depending on what the law proscribes at the time.

The benefits of crime for society, however, can be more subtle than the fulfillment of formally prohibited individual appetites. Whyte's classic studies show that the rackets become a source of integration in a low-income area and offer a path of upward social mobility (1943, 1958). Merton (1968:185-248), Cloward and Ohlin (1960), and others have argued that members of deprived groups seek illegitimate means to socially approved ends when they lack the opportunity for access to legitimate means. Thus, crime can serve as a route to success, when legitimate routes like a college education are unavailable. From a different perspective, Erikson (1962, 1966) has followed Durkheim's (1958) principle that crime is a part of all healthy societies and has set forth the general proposition that deviance helps a society maintain its boundaries. Through the example of his behavior, the deviant stands as a contrast to the range of activity a community defines as acceptable.

Medical sociologists have recognized for some time that illness, like crime, is a form of deviance. In his classic analysis of the sick role, Parsons has conceptualized illness largely as a problem in social control (1951:312-313, 428-479). The physician, in this view, becomes an agent of social control who certifies illness and either permits or restricts entry into the sick role. As Cumming has shown, the physician acts as part of a "system of social regulation"; the doctor's role differs mainly in degree from that of the clergyman, social worker, or policeman (1968). Fox has discussed the "latent social control functions" of the physician, who "sorts out 'malingerers' "—denying them the "exonerations of sickness"—and sets in motion a therapeutic process to return those certified as ill to their "full-scale participation" in society (1968). Mechanic has introduced his comprehensive review of medical sociology by viewing disease, and especially "illness behavior," as a form of deviance (1968:15-48). In his theoretical analysis and critique of professionalism, Freidson has developed a typology of diseases which reflect varying degrees of deviance (1970a: 205-243). Kasl and Cobb have characterized the sick role as one of a number of possible deviant reactions to strain in the social system (1966). Scheff (1966), Goffman (1961:127 ff.), and Szasz (1961, 1963) have shown that in decisions about commitment to mental hospitals, psychiatrists enforce conventional rules of appropriate versus deviant social behavior. Nearly a century ago, Samuel Butler extended the similarities between illness and crime to a satirical conclusion: ". . . in that country if a man falls into ill health, or catches any disorder, or fails bodily in any way before he is seventy years old, he is tried before a jury of his countrymen, and if convicted is held up to public scorn and sentenced more or less severely as the case may be" (1961:67).

In these writings we can follow two theoretical strands. First, crime and related forms of deviance can make beneficial contributions to society. Second, illness is a form of deviance, controlled through the patterning of the sick role. From this perspective it is surprising that the following question seldom is asked: Does it make any sense to assert that illness, or more especially the adoption of the sick role, is a natural and even beneficial part of social life? This question applies Erikson's more general problem— ". . . does it make any sense to assert that deviant forms of behavior are a natural and even beneficial part of social life?" (1966:5)— to the specific problem of the sick role.

THEORETICAL CONSIDERATIONS

The latent functions of the sick role   The central theme in this section is that the sick role contributes to social stability in a wide variety of institutional settings. This stabilizing effect may be viewed as a "latent function."

The sick role provides a controllable form of deviance which mitigates potentially disruptive conflicts between personality needs and the social system's role demands. Although details vary in each institutional setting, the sick role is found to serve stabilizing functions in the family, mental hospital, totalitarian state, penal institution, armed forces, and Selective Service System. In all these settings, adoption of the sick role relieves strains which otherwise could become a focus of dissatisfaction, conflict, and change. To the extent that it fosters social stability and defuses potential opposition, the sick role's effects tend to be conservative and, perhaps in some cases, counterrevolutionary.

Nowadays sociologists often are abashed when they use the theoretical perspective of functionalism. For example, Erikson vividly illustrates the "beneficial part" of deviance in Puritan society but apologetically distinguishes this from "functions":

> If our culture has supported a steady flow of deviation throughout long periods of historical change, the rules which apply to any kind of evolutionary thinking would suggest that strong forces must be at work to keep the flow intact—and this because it contributes in some important way to the survival of the culture as a whole. This does not furnish us with sufficient warrant to declare that deviance is "functional" (in any of the senses of the term), but it should certainly make us wary of the assumption so often made in sociological circles that any well-structured society is somehow designed to prevent deviant behavior from occurring (1966:18).

The benefits of deviance derive, according to Erikson, from its contribution to the "survival" of the culture as a whole. Does this view differ from Merton's (1968:117) definition of functions as the "objective consequences" of a behavioral pattern which contribute to the "adjustment or adaptation" of a system of action? Erikson's "benefits of deviance" to "survival" seem to be, in Merton's terms, "objective consequences" which contribute to "adjustment or adaptation." It appears that different words here refer to the same thing.

In many functional analyses the "objective consequences" (Merton's terms) have not been especially objective. The labeling of behavioral patterns as functional frequently becomes an interpretive exercise bearing a tenuous relation to empirical data. To invoke Popper's famous criterion, claims of functionality often lack the attribute of falsifiability; they cannot be disproved by data (Popper, 1959; Nagel, 1961; Homans, 1964). Any behavioral pattern can become the object of functional interpretation; if it were not somehow functional, it would not persist. The largely speculative nature of many functional analyses may account for the present disrepute into which functionalism has fallen.

There is, in our opinion, no wholly satisfactory methodological solution to this problem. In this chapter we suggest several ways in which adoption of the sick role can contribute to the stability of social institutions, thus serving a latent function. The theoretical perspective is Merton's (1968: 117): *the sick role serves a latent function in a social system to the extent that its objective consequences (a) contribute to the system's adjustment or adaptation and (b) are neither intended nor consciously recognized by those who adopt the sick role.* None of the propositions we discuss is fully falsifiable. It cannot be said, for example, that if access to the sick role were severely limited, certain institutions like prisons, the armed forces and the Selective Service System would not survive. On the other hand, there is evidence that adoption of the sick role is functional in maintaining all these institutions. A comparative perspective of these institutions may enhance our understanding of the latent functions of the sick role in Weber's sense (Weber, 1964). But since these ideas are not fully falsifiable, they must remain suggestive rather than conclusive.[1]

Variable criteria for physicians' certification of illness The latent functions of the sick role depend on the existence within a social system of professionals who control access to the role. These professionals permit adoption of the sick role by certifying illness under certain circumstances. However, partly because of the potentially disruptive effects of widespread adoption of the sick role, they restrict access according to unique criteria within each institutional setting. The criteria of certification must be so ill-defined that they can be stretched or manipulated within limits determined by institutional requirements.

The relationship between physiologic state and the differential patterning of the sick role can be considered schematically in Figure 3. In a given institutional setting, physicians evaluate a range of overt complaints, relative to physiologic disturbance, as appropriate for adoption of the sick role. Increasing complaints should reflect increasing physiologic disturbance, and variation in complaints (related to age, ethnicity, social class, etc.) can occur only within a range of appropriate sick role behavior. The restrictiveness of criteria for certification of illness depends on institutional setting. It might be predicted that the range of behavior satisfactory for certification in some institutions, such as the armed forces, would be narrower than in other institutions, such as prisons; these relationships are depicted in Figure 3 as a more limited range of appropriate sick role behavior in Institution A as compared to Institution B. Overt complaints in excess of the institutionally appropriate range of sick role behavior are considered "malingering"; minimization or denial of symptoms relative to physiologic disturbance is viewed as "stoicism." It should be noted that the scope of behavior defined as malingering or stoicism also varies with institutional setting. As the range of appropriate sick role behavior narrows, the incidence of behavior judged to reflect malingering or stoicism would increase.

According to the unique criteria of the institutional settings in which they work, physicians may permit access to the sick role, encourage stoicism, or denounce malingering—in the latter case, denying access to the sick role. The latent functions of the sick role thus depend on

1. Recent analyses of public welfare systems in Europe and the United States and of health care in Israel have employed similar functional perspectives (Piven and Cloward, 1971; Shuval, 1970).The methodological and ideological problems of functional analysis are also receiving more constructive critical attention (Gans, 1972).

Figure 3. Hypothetical relationship between physiologic disturbance and overt complaints appropriate for adoption of the sick role in different institutional settings

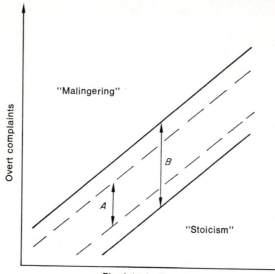

Source: "Latent Functions of the Sick Role in Various Institutional Settings" by Howard Waitzkin, in Social Science and Medicine 5 (1971): 47. Reprinted courtesy of Pergamon Press. We are indebted to Charles E. Lewis for suggesting the pictorial presentation of these concepts.

A = appropriate sick role behavior in institution A
B = appropriate sick role behavior in institution B

physicians' application of decision-making criteria which vary in different institutional settings. Other writers, notably Gordon (1966), have emphasized that the sick role comprises a more variable range of behavior than Parsons described in his classic analysis (1951). It is the institutional variability in criteria for adoption of the sick role which we emphasize here.

Latent functions and secondary gain   One of our purposes in this chapter is to reconcile the concept of "secondary gain" as it is employed in psychosomatic medicine and medical sociology with the concept of "latent function." There are two distinct levels at which secondary gain can be conceptualized. Secondary gain from adoption of the sick role can accrue to the *individual,* since the sick role can satisfy certain personality needs which otherwise would go unfulfilled. For example, an individual with unsatisfied needs for nurturance or attention might find that the sick role offers attractive psychological benfits. In addition, entry into the sick role can provide secondary gain to the *social system* of which the sick individual is a member. When potentially disruptive strains exist in the social system, the assumption of the sick role by one of its members can stabilize role relationships and thereby contribute to the social system's survival.

Inkeles' theoretical framework elucidates the secondary gain which the sick role can contribute to both personality and social system. According to Inkeles, every social system makes certain role demands of its members. Moreover, at the level of personality, each individual possesses a number of psychological needs. The adjustment and performance of both social system and individual, Inkeles concludes, depends on the articulation between personality needs and role demands (1963).

When conflict arises between personality needs and role demands, the sick role provides one mechanism by which this conflict can be resolved. The sick role allows the individual to deviate from normal role demands and, by the attention and nurturance one is likely to receive, to satisfy certain personality needs. These outcomes represent secondary gain *to the individual.* While the sick role allows a limited degree of deviance, however, it is a form of deviance which can be carefully controlled without major social disruption. By providing a controllable, nondisruptive mode of deviance when conflicts arise between personality needs and role demands, the sick role helps preserve social stability and thus offers secondary gain *to the social system.* From this latter viewpoint, secondary gain from the sick role is a contribution to the social system's adjustment or adaptation which is not intended or recognized by those who assume the sick role. *Secondary gain at the level of the social system is therefore a type of latent function,* as defined above. To summarize: the sick role can yield secondary gain to the individual and to the social system. In the latter case, secondary gain is equivalent to what we have called a latent function of the sick role.[2]

For analysis in this chapter, we have selected a number of institutional settings in which conflicts between role demands and personality needs can become severe. In each case the sick role appears to offer secondary gain—i.e. serves latent functions—for the social system. It is the stabilizing functions of the sick role *at the level of the social system* which we emphasize. Because perspectives on the family, mental hospital, and totalitarian state are available from previous research, we discuss these institutional settings chiefly as a selective review of available literature. Then we concentrate on the prison, armed forces, and the military draft for more detailed analysis. Other institutional settings than those analyzed here are also relevant and are discussed briefly in conclusion.

2. Since we consider the gains from the sick role to both the individual and the social system, our perspective incorporates elements of social psychological (cf. Malinowski, 1926, 1939) and sociological (Radcliffe-Brown, 1935, 1948) functionalism. A detailed exposition of this traditional distinction in functionalist theory and its historical nuances, however, is beyond the scope of our discussion.

PREVIOUS RESEARCH

The family Families usually pull together in times of crisis. Although the stabilizing function of acute illness is evident, some families also establish longterm relationships based on chronic impairment or disease. Vogel and Bell have shown that the emotionally disturbed child can function as the family scapegoat, allowing parents to channel tensions which otherwise would destroy family life (1968). For example, a mother who resents her husband's lack of achievement in work may select as a scapegoat that child who most resembles the father in appearance or who shows unsatisfactory achievement in school. The mother chooses some symptom and helps to maintain it, thus reinforcing the child's adoption of the sick role. Although she may criticize and sometimes even punish the child, she also supports in subtle ways the persistence of the behavior. The mother of a child with enuresis may reprimand the child intermittently but also may continue to put a rubber sheet on the bed and to buy special night clothes in case the child wets: "While the explanation given for this inconsistency was that he [the parent] wanted to teach the desired behavior without being 'too hard on the child,' its latent function was to prevent the child from consistently living up to the ostensibly desired behavior and to preserve the disliked behavior" (Vogel and Bell, 1968:421). Through this scapegoating process, parents are able to control their own interpersonal conflicts by projecting them onto one of the children. As a result, the family maintains its stability while the child's problem persists.

Bursten and D'Esopo's work demonstrates that in certain families similar underlying conflicts result in the maintenance of persisting patterns of illness in adults (1965). Such families promote a "stable equilibrium" by obliging a particular family member to remain sick. For example, "a wife may express concern, sympathy, overprotectiveness as if she wanted him [her husband] to improve, but at the same time she may convey to him the underlying feeling that sickness is what is expected" (Bursten and D'Esopo, 1965:406). Through the sick role, these families can avoid explicit consideration of potentially disruptive tensions. In such families there is a broad range of overt complaints, relative to physiologic disturbance, which is appropriate for adoption of the sick role.

As Parsons and Fox have pointed out, the modern urban family experiences unique strains which are intimately related to the adoption of the sick role. Because the nuclear family has become isolated from the emotional supports of extended kinship relations, it has become particularly vulnerable to these strains. The sick role can provide an escape from the mother's "heavy 'human relations management'" responsibilities or from the father's obligations within the occupational structure (Parsons and Fox, 1952). In this perspective, the sick role serves as a temporary safety valve, which allows the family to protect itself from intermittent pressures which otherwise could prove overwhelming.

Finally, some families can benefit from the sick role in more tangible ways. Most departments of public welfare specify that certain items may be provided to welfare recipients if a physician certifies a family's need for such items. For example, welfare recipients in Massachusetts may not receive payments for telephones unless they can show some special need for it:

> Recipients may have various non-basic or special needs which are essential to their welfare. These items shall be allowed in accordance with the Standards of Assistance as determined by investigation or re-investigation. In addition to those outlined below other needs that shall be provided, as required on a casework basis, are laundry, household chores, telephone, special diets, etc. (Commonwealth of Massachusetts, 1970).

Welfare recipients know that certification of need by a physician will result in their receiving a telephone. They also know that a telephone has become a necessity for families trying to survive on low incomes in cities. When they or their children are sick, they often ask the attending physician to write a letter to the welfare department, stating the need for a telephone. Occasionally, they ask the physician to certify need even when there is no current illness which the physician is treating (Children's Hospital Medical Center, 1970). Because of the welfare system's regulations, the sick role can bring material possessions without which the family's integrity would be more difficult to maintain.

The mental hospital   Although mental hospitals have a certain latitude in labeling patients as healthy or ill, the tendency is toward designating them as ill (Scheff, 1966; Goffman, 1961). Staff members of mental hospitals illustrate this tendency by their entries in patients' case records. As Goffman points out, the dossier shows that staff members base their treatment of patients upon their diagnoses and a psychiatric view of their past:

> The dossier is apparently not regularly used, however, to record occasions when the patient showed capacity to cope honorably and effectively with difficult life situations. Nor is the case record typically used to provide a rough average or sampling of his past conduct. One of its purposes is to show the ways in which the patient is "sick" and the reasons why it was right to commit him and is right to keep him committed; and this is done by extracting from his whole life course a list of those incidents that have or might have had "symptomatic" significance (1961: 155–156).

Behavior labeled as appropriate outside the mental hospital tends to become inappropriate inside, as is evident from the verbatim transcriptions of case records reported by Goffman:

> "The patient denied any heterosexual experiences nor could one trick her into admitting that she had ever been pregnant or into any kind of sexual indulgence, denying masturbation as well. . . . Even with considerable pressure she was unwilling to engage in any projection of paranoid mechanisms. . . . No psychotic content could be elicited at this time" (1961:157).

Although the public goal of the mental hospital is to help patients get well, institutionalized expectations of staff members seem to demand that within the hospital patients be sick. Thus there appears to be a broad range of behavior defined as consistent with adoption of the sick role in the mental hospital.

The staff of the mental hospital expect the patient to manifest symptoms of illness. The patient may resist these expectations and may disagree with the label of psychic disturbance. But staff members stand to gain from the patient's uncomplaining adoption of the sick role. Goffman states:

> If both the custodial and psychiatric factions are to get him to cooperate in the various psychiatric treatments, then it will be useful to disabuse him of his view of their purposes, and cause him to appreciate that they know what they are doing, and are doing what is best for him. In brief, the difficulties caused by a patient are closely tied to his version of what has been happening to him, and if cooperation is to be secured, it helps if this version is discredited. The patient must "insightfully" come to take, or affect to take, the hospital's view of himself (1961:154–155).

The patient's adoption of the sick role with minimal resistance serves a latent function by allowing the mental hospital to avoid conflict. To the extent that reduction of conflict is an institutional goal, the mental hospital benefits from the patient's ready acceptance of the sick role.

Although one may not consider oneself sick for some time, a patient learns that the easiest way to get along in the institution is to enter fully into the sick role and to display the signs of mental illness which others expect. With this insight, the patient develops and perhaps exaggerates the display of symptoms, so that staff members realistically see something to treat:

> The patient is thus often persuaded by the logic of psychiatric institutions to attempt to engineer validation in the role this society provides for the medical patient—in which, to be sure, distinctly psychotic patients are presumed to belong. To establish his eligibility for this conventional role, the mental patient must negotiate, using his illness as an instrumentality. He must present illness to others in a form which they recognize as legitimate, perhaps even exaggerating his portrayal of those behaviors which qualify medical patients for their role. In having to do so, the argument continues, he is often left with little choice but to become sicker or more chronically sick (Erikson, 1957:264).

Because of the expectations of the social system, the mental patient must act as though he or she needs treatment.

An individual's adoption of the sick role in adjusting to the mental hospital implies that recovery, which involves leaving the sick role, becomes problematic. On the one hand the patient must play the sick role to establish a stable position in the institution. On the other hand, if one is to recover, one's behavior must change to a form which is inappropriate vis-a-vis the institutional expectations of the mental hospital. Erikson describes the countervailing pressures which stand in the way of recovery:

. . . when the patient has to seek definition as acutely ill and helpless in order to achieve a measure of public validation for his illness—and simultaneously has to use all his remaining strengths to struggle against that illness—a dilemma is posed which he may resolve by simply giving up the struggle altogether and submerging himself in the sick definition permanently (1957:271).

Although adoption of the sick role helps minimize conflict in the mental hospital, the resulting counter-pressures create a situation in which passage from the sick role is difficult.

The totalitarian state　A totalitarian state places strict demands on individual action. Each person occupies a role defined as essential in the social system and is expected to work toward maximum productivity. In order to maintain the uniformity of its standards, the totalitarian state must control deviance carefully. During the Stalinist regime in the Soviet Union, each individual was expected to work regularly and consistently on the job, contributing to the over-all production of the state. Illness, certified by a physician, provided the only way an individual legitimately could be excused from responsibilities in production. Persons with a variety of reasons to miss work resorted to the sick role. In the totalitarian state the sick role permitted limited deviant behavior and thereby satisfied certain needs whose continued frustration might have threatened the stability of the regime. The range of overt complaints appropriate for adoption of the sick role, however, was quite narrow.

If an individual during the Stalinist period wished a certificate of illness to obtain an excuse from work, he or she had to consult a physician authorized by the government to issue such certificates. As Field's studies have shown, workers could use several different techniques designed to obtain certification of illness from authorized physicians, including simulation of symptoms and signs (1953, 1957, 1967). As an alternative approach, an individual could consult a physician and simply request a medical certificate, without presenting any symptoms of illness. In this case one could offer the physician a story—most likely concerning the necessity of missing work to attend to the needs of one's family—which would arouse pity or sympathy. A third possibility, in addition to producing artificial symptoms and signs and using stories to arouse pity, involved a person whose symptoms were real and not simulated. A worker experiencing objective symptoms often sought the care of a physician who was known personally but who was unauthorized to issue medical certificates. Such a patient might approach an authorized physician, requesting a medical certificate but no medical attention.

The physician's standing among political and professional superiors in the Stalinist period depended largely on how quickly his or her patients returned to their active responsibilities in the occupational system. (As we shall discuss shortly, a similar prestige system operates in the armed forces.) On the other hand the patient in the Soviet system was free to denounce a physician by writing critical letters to the editor of newspapers. Because of these cross-pressures, contact between physicians and patients was marked by mutual suspicion. Physicians were required to ascertain whether patients were simulating their symptoms. Patients, some of whom actually experienced the symptoms they reported, had to make a great effort to convince physicians that their incapacity was real. With these cross-pressures, trust between doctor and patient broke down.

Convalescence was shortened in the Soviet system. Because requirements for production did not permit an extended period of recovery, the physician limited medical certification to the shortest possible period of time. During the Stalinist regime illness was to be certified every three days if an individual continued to occupy the sick role.

Nevertheless, when individuals experience personal problems or desires which motivate them to miss work, the sick role remains available in a totalitarian state. Frustration of individual wants, when severe and prolonged, can lead to revolt against the regime. By allowing deviance within the carefully controlled framework of the sick role, the totalitarian state helps protect its own stability.

THE PENAL INSTITUTION

Medical care in the Mettray infirmary was no better than it is here . . . Nevertheless, the infirmary was a paradise for us.—Jean Genet, **Miracle of the Rose** *(1966:271).*

Prisons face unique problems of deviance and social control. As Sykes demonstrates, penal institutions tend to work out the problem of social control by granting a large measure of unofficial control to the inmates themselves:

> *. . . the unofficial control of the prison by the inmates oriented to the theme of inmate cohesion is slipped into more easily because exploitation, conflict among prisoners, and aggression against custodians is curbed by the inmates themselves. Both the guard and the inmate desire an "easy bit" and both want to keep things from being "all shook up" (1958:128).*

Although most jails and prisons undergo periods of clamping down, inmates generally can develop an underlife which makes their stay in the institution more bearable. One aspect of this underlife is the sick role, which the social system of the penal institution patterns in a characteristic way. The sick role represents a controlled form of deviance, which prisons can permit with a certain latitude. By allowing inmates to adopt the sick role almost at will, prisons provide a legitimate outlet for deviant behavior—which, if expressed in other forms, could seriously threaten institutional stability. It might be added, however, that although entry into the sick role is not tightly restricted, medical care in prisons is usually extremely poor in quality, as will be described. In a penal institution, the range of behavior appropriate for adoption of the sick role is wider than in the totalitarian state or, as we shall discuss, the armed forces.

The following observations emerged from a four-month field study of sick call behavior in an urban men's penal institution (referred to here as "City Jail") which was conducted in 1967. The study involved observations of actual sick calls at the hospital attached to the institution; focused interviews with inmates, physicians who worked at the hospital, nurses, guards, and other officials; and observations of living and working conditions in the cell blocks and dormitories (Waitzkin, 1969).

To make the transition to the sick role in City Jail, an individual may experience objective symptoms, or he may not. Reporting on sick call does not require the display of observable signs. One merely need say that he wishes to report on sick call, and he is allowed to do so. Discouragement of a prisoner's reporting on sick call, by either guards or fellow inmates, was not observed at any time in the field study.

Several aspects of the social system, however, can influence whether one actually experiences symptoms. For example, difficulties can arise from communal living. A large number of inmates reporting on sick call at City Jail complain of sleeplessness. Insomnia and chronic headaches may develop largely because of the number of individuals who must live in close proximity. In addition, "shortitis" is a common malady in City Jail. An inmate who has become adjusted to institutional life may face his release with considerable apprehension. Such an individual, who may be bothered by insomnia, headaches, the jitters, or other problems, may report on sick call frequently during his final weeks in jail. Thus, one man reporting on sick call said that he needed something to help him sleep at night; he had only seventeen more days to do and had—as he put it—shortitis. Another man, complaining of a runny nose, asked to be granted a "lay in" in the hospital attached to the institution. He told the physician, "I'm getting out next week, and I don't want to get messed up." This meant that he wanted to avoid getting into trouble, which would extend his sentence, and that a stay in the hospital would help him keep in line.

Other inmates in City Jail develop symptoms and adopt the sick role because of personal psychological needs which the social system does not fulfill in other ways. Many individuals confined in penal institutions feel a sense of rejection by the outside world. In some cases they considered their family life unsatisfactory before they entered prison; in other cases family or friends drift away from inmates while they are in jail. One of the few places in the social system of the penal institution which provides the inmate with some sense of being cared for is the medical facility. One sergeant who supervises a dormitory in City Jail expressed the opinion that many inmates develop symptoms and report on sick call to fulfill such psychological needs:

Sick call is good. These things are a must. It's a psychological thing anyway. A lot of young ones, on the outside, have no father, no mother, aren't wanted. [Sick call] makes them think people do care for them.

Lydston, a physician working in British prisons at the turn of the century, recognized similar psychological benefits of illness in prison life:

> [Malingering in the use of sick call arises from] a craving for sympathy. . . . The intensification of the ego on the part of the criminal is a further explantation, in that it leads him to believe in himself as an object of solicitude, or, at least, of interest on the part of others (1911:387).

Institutionalized norms governing conduct in prisons militate against psychological support and nurturance. Guards' behavior must be tough, even if they inwardly emphathize with the prisoners' condition. Similarly, norms of toughness prevail among inmates themselves; overt expression of psychological needs reduce one's status. The sick role permits satisfaction of these needs for the individual while preserving the institution's norms of appropriate behavior.

In addition to the real psychological and physical symptoms sometimes experienced by inmates, the underlife of City Jail can motivate inmates to report on sick call. In this case the individual need not necessarily have experienced objective symptoms; simulation of symptoms is sufficient to enter the sick role. The underlife of a penal institution typically is characterized not by inactivity and boredom, but—as a physician attached to City Jail put it—by "wheeling and dealing." The sick role permits the development of stable but informal social networks, which the penal institution formally prohibits. To the extent that it supports these informal networks, the sick role allows limited deviance and the fulfillment of needs whose frustration might lead to conflict within the institution.

Inmates within the institution constantly try to keep in touch with each other. Through such contact they make life more interesting and enjoyable for themselves. Two buddies, housed in different parts of City Jail, may arrange to report on sick call the same morning. Norman describes a similar use of sick call by inmates of a British prison:

> The sick parade is the biggest giggle you know, if there is twenty men on the sick list may be one of them has got something wrong with them maybe, most of the chaps on the sick parade either go because they don't feel like going to work that morning or they arrange with someone they want to see, who is in another hall to go sick as well. Which is one of the only ways of being sure of making a meet, and keeping it. In some of the very big nicks you can have a mate in one hall and you are in another and it is quite possible that you may not see him or he you the whole time you are there, even if you are both there for years. So you have to make these sort of arrangements so that you can (1958:44).

Such meetings permit buddies in City Jail to discuss many topics of mutual interest—especially information from outside the institution which one buddy might have received from a visitor.

Sick call in City Jail also serves as a convenient meeting place for sexual activity. Inmates whose homosexuality becomes evident to the staff are segregated into a special dormitory. During their hours in the dormitory, a guard supervises them trying to prevent sexual liaison. These men work together in the laundry, and there, too, little chance for sexual contact arises. Supervision during sick call is not as strict. While the physician sees a group of patients, the rest wait in the hallway outside the examining room. During this time it is possible for two men to leave the group without being noticed and to enter one of the washrooms or broom closets in the hallway. After a few minutes together, they can return to the rest of the group.

Gathering for sick call furthermore provides a central exchange point for the delivery of notes (known as "kites") to other parts of City Jail. Censorship discourages written contact between inmates along formal channels. At sick call inmates can pass notes to men they meet from other parts of the institution, or they can give notes to an orderly or runner. The latter are inmates who have obtained positions of trust; orderlies work at the medical facility and runners deliver minor messages for staff members in various buildings of the institutional complex. By pocketing a note, an orderly or runner later can deliver it to the intended recipient. Although the social system formally limits many modes of communication among inmates, sick call offers an informal channel.

Another benefit of the sick role in City Jail is that it provides inmates with certain commodities which the institution cannot legitimately offer on a regular basis. Officials realize, on the other hand, that the demand for the commodities is high and that prisoners might use force against each other to obtain them if they were not available through other mechanisms. By distributing these products to inmates who adopt the sick role, the prison satisfies demand without doing so as a matter of policy.

For example, it is very easy to obtain some types of drugs as a result of reporting on sick call. Formerly, the physician supervising sick call at City Jail dispensed a number of pills, to be taken at specified intervals. More recently, it has been found that inmates have hoarded pills, rather than taking them as instructed. As a result, the pills now are sent from the dispensary to the officer in charge of the inmate's dormitory or cell block. He is supposed to give the inmate a pill as directed and to make sure the inmate swallows the pill in his presence. However, it is still possible for an inmate to "palm" the pill or to hold it in his cheek, saving it along with other pills prescribed for him. The purposes of hoarding pills are twofold. First, an inmate who has saved his pills can take a large number at once. Inmates use this technique to "get high," an experience of stimulation which is greatly valued. Second, a supply of pills can become an article of exchange (much like money or cigarettes in other contexts). An inmate can buy some goods on his weekly visit to the commissary. But this takes money, and few inmates have much money deposited for them in their institutional accounts. Therefore, if an inmate with a supply of pills knows another inmate with a desired article or with money on deposit, and if the other inmate sees the value of getting high, they can make an exchange.

In addition to pills, an inmate who has a rash or acne usually can obtain some kind of ointment for the skin. Because it is possible to use ointment to grease one's body so that it is more difficult to be held by guards, officials in penal institutions traditionally have limited the dispensation of ointments. Inmates often use the small amounts of ointment they can receive for other than medicinal purposes. For example, certain cosmetic agents are popular in the outside world but are unavailable in prison. As a result some prisoners try to get ointment to use as hair oil. For others ointment sometimes can serve as a sexual lubricant. A physician working in City Jail commented: "There are a lot of perverts in this place. If I prescribe ointment, they can use it for perverse homosexuality." Nevertheless, this physican provided small tubes of ointment to a number of patients with mild skin rashes. In this way the sick role permits the prison to meet inmates' demand for commodities which are formally unavailable in the institutional economy.

Inmates also gain in more obvious ways from adopting the sick role. If a prisoner wants to avoid work on a given morning, reporting on sick call results in an automatic excuse from his prison job. Or, if life occasionally becomes excessively monotonous, sick call provides a break in routine through a trip to the hospital, which is located in a different building from the cell blocks and dormitories. There is strong evidence that many inmates use sick call in these ways. It was found that 44 percent of a random sample of inmates in City Jail reported on sick call two times or more in a three-month period. This figure is over two times as large as the percentage of Army men who reported on sick call twice or more in a much longer period of time—the three-year period from 1952 to 1955 (Harris and Little, 1957). The vast majority of cases seen in sick call involve minor reported symptomatology, which requires no further medical attention. The physician who supervises sick call claimed that only about one-third of the men he sees have physical reasons for reporting on sick call.

That sick call provides nonmedical benefits for inmates is reflected in the fact that the number of inmates reporting on sick call in City Jail was halved when the superintendent ruled that all men on sick call must miss breakfast. Apparently the attractiveness of the sick role diminished when a person had to lose a meal in order to adopt the role. Lydston, writing in 1911, reported success with a similar method:

> I finally hit upon the expedient of having the sick call at dinner time. The success of the experiment was astounding, as evidenced by the fact that, whereas 180 men appeared at sick call the day previous, there were only twelve in line on the first day of the experiment. The latter number is about the average number that presented themselves during the rest of my term of service. As my orderly expressed it, they couldn't "stand the smell of the soup" (1911:388).

These observations indicate that the sick role is a form of deviance which the penal institution tolerates to a limited extent, perhaps because it is easier to control than other forms of deviance. In this sense, the sick role serves as a "buffer" which mediates between the demands of the social system and the needs of the individual. Inmates can enter the sick role and make gains which the social system allows the sick but not the well.

Treatment at City Jail is brief and perfunctory. During sick call a single physician generally sees about thirty inmates in approximately one and one-half hours. This means that on the average, consultation lasts about three minutes. For the majority of these patients, treatment consists of a limited supply of drugs which they are supposed to consume on the day they report on sick call and possibly the day after. In one sick call, the physician saw twenty-four inmates. For twenty-one of these, he prescribed a small supply of some kind of pill. Two men received a salve for a rash on the body. Five were referred to clinics in the hospital for further attention to medical problems. During a second sick call, the physician saw thirty-one inmates. Twenty-two of these received a prescription for pills, four obtained an ointment, and eight were referred to other clinics.

In processing the men on sick call, the physician sat behind a desk and called one inmate at a time. Each inmate stood before the desk and described his symptoms. For colds, headaches, sleeplessness, and digestive problems, the symptoms most frequently presented, the physician remained seated, wrote out a prescription which was to be sent to the dispensary, and told the inmate he would receive medicine in his cell block or dormitory. Only when a person described a definite physical problem—a rash, corns on the feet, difficulties with a gunshot wound in the stomach, or psoriasis—did the physician rise from his seat to examine the inmate more carefully.

The inmate's actual encounter with the physician is thus largely symbolic. The limited dosage of a drug is a symbol that the institution has fulfilled its responsibility for the health of inmates. As far as the institution is concerned, the patient's illness ends when he has swallowed his pill or applied his ointment. If an individual wants to adopt the sick role again (for example, if he wants more pills or ointment), he must report on sick call again. The physician sees his own role essentially as a screening agent who refers serious medical problems to other clinics and satisfies the majority of inmates on sick call with a small dosage of a mild drug.

When questioned about his prescriptions, one physician working at City Jail stated that he gives aspirin for headaches, antitussives and aspirin for colds, antacids for stomach problems, and analgesics for muscular aches and pains. Yet he recognized most of the drugs he prescribes are mainly significant for their symbolic meaning—i.e., that the institution does something about the inmates' health—rather than for their medicinal effect. He stated:

> Much of the stuff I prescribe is for symptomatic relief. In my mind I know a patient doesn't need anything. In private practice I'd tell a patient there's nothing wrong—just rest up. But in an institution, it's different, and you can't just give a lay-in [admit an inmate to the hospital].

Knowing that most inmates on sick call are not there for strictly physical reasons, the physician also knows that he must respond in some way to the inmates' complaints. As a nurse pointed out, inmates who are released from a public institution can create a scandal by complaining about medical services within the institution. Thus the social system requires that each inmate who adopts the sick role obtain a response, albeit a symbolic response, from the physician.

For the few inmates who are referred from sick call to other clinics, treatment continues. For the majority, however, the sick role ends when they consume the limited number of pills which have been prescribed. The institution does not initiate a follow-up to make sure an individual has recovered. If the sick role has satisfied his needs, he simply drops the issue. As indicated by the low rate of repeaters to successive sick calls (approximately 1 to 2 percent at City Jail), this seems to be the case most of the time. If not satisfied, the inmate must enter the sick role again, submitting his name for sick call, recounting his problem to the physician, and again receiving his small dosage of medication. By adopting the sick role, the prisoner can deviate temporarily within carefully controlled limits and in a manner which does not jeopardize the prison's stability.

THE ARMED FORCES

Passive-dependent behavior is met with an aloof attitude and a harsh confrontation. Passive-aggressive behavior is laughed at and supplementary calisthenics are matter of factly ordered for all obstructionism. These techniques quickly and effectively communicate to the recruit that appropriate limits will be maintained regardless of his behavior.— J. C. Dodgen and J. B. Brickman, "The psychotherapy of maladjusted Marine recruits" (1967:916).

The armed forces adopt military efficiency as a primary goal. Each individual within the social system comprising the armed forces has a role to play in working toward this goal. The system places strenuous demands on the individual, who knows that he is expected to be more concerned with the welfare of the system than with his own. Similarly, according to the norms governing provision of medical care in the armed forces, physicians are to direct their efforts primarily toward preserving the military efficiency of the entire combat unit and secondarily toward maintaining the health of the individual soldier. The U.S. Army Field Manual states these norms explicity:

The mission of the medical services in a theater of operations is to contribute to the success of the military effort through—(a) Conserving manpower. Military strength is preserved by seeing that only the fit take the field, by the protection of troops against unnecessary hazards to health and efficiency, and by the effective care and early return to duty. (b) Preventing adverse effects of unevacuated casualties on combat efficiency. Casualties within any combat unit restrict its movement. Lack of care and proper evacuation reduces the soldier's willingness to take necessary risks (U.S. Army, 1959).

Within this context both doctor and patient are aware of the possible conflicts which can arise between the individual's physical and psychological needs and the social system's demands.

The armed forces permit deviance only within narrowly defined limits.

As might be expected, an individual who cannot cope with or conform to the demands of the system looks for an escape route. As Little points out, the sick role is the only authorized route by which an individual can gain exemption from his usual obligations (1956). It permits the soldier who cannot meet the system's demands to deviate within limits. In addition, the sick role formally isolates the deviant soldier from his peers and assures that his exemption from responsibilities does not interfere with the activities of the rest of his unit. Because it provides a buffer which allows limited individual deviance while maintaining efficiency and uniformity of standards in the larger group, the sick role serves a stabilizing function for both the individual and the social system.

Nevertheless, the range of behavior appropriate for adoption of the sick role is narrow, especially in basic training, but also in other areas of military life. A medical officer must legitimate an individual's adoption of the sick role. Thus an individual cannot "be sick" in the armed forces without consulting the prescribed medical authority. As can be inferred from Schneider's analysis of basic training, the decision to seek medical attention is probably a personal one, without much "lay" discussion with one's peers (Schneider, 1964; cf. Freidson, 1961). This is because group norms discourage the adoption of the sick role and effectively cut off the individual who does assume the role from the rest of the group:

> The sick man is then actively despised and aggressed against; he is brushed from the field. He retires, securing himself with the previously accepted sanction that the sick cannot be expected to do things, and he does not do them. He continues to define the situation as he had at the outset and only gradually abandons his attempts to force his definition of the situation onto the others (Schneider, 1964:389).

Apparently the sanctions of the group create an effective deterrent which prevents widespread deviance through the adoption of the sick role. Such a conclusion seems warranted by Harris and Little's finding that few men avail themselves of the sick role as an escape route. Within a population of over 2200 men in the Far East between 1952 and 1955, 62 percent never went on sick call, 19 percent went once, 13 percent went two or three times, 5 percent four to six times, and 3 percent more than seven times (Harris and Little, 1957:175). (As previously mentioned, these figures indicate a much lower utilization of sick call than in the penal institution which was studied.) Because of the pressure of group norms, the social system appears to restrict consultation with the medical officer but still permits a small proportion of soldiers to adopt the sick role relatively frequently.

While he occupies the sick role, the individual is isolated from his unit and exempted from his usual duties. As Little puts it, "one 'had it made' when admitted to the hospital" (1956:23). However, the sick soldier undergoes continuing pressure to give up the sick role and to return to his duties. This pressure comes mainly from the medical officer, whose own status within the military organization depends on how quickly the patient's stay in the hospital comes to an end. Little points out that the medical officer's superiors judge his technical competence on the basis of his success in "limiting the number of persons who could be legitimately designed as 'sick'" (1956:24).

Even an individual who enters the sick role because of psychological difficulties can expect pressure from medical authorities to relinquish the sick role as soon as possible. As Bushard states, the Army has been able to limit the assumption of the sick role by adopting the policy that soldiers with emotional problems not be exempted from their duties:

> Every effort is made to avoid interruption of training. Hospitalization is avoided if at all possible, as is the patient's being taken for any significant period of time from actual, if impaired, participation in military routine . . . Physical separation of the patient from the scene of his difficulties is accompanied most frequently by his indulging in the hope of not having to return (1957:440–441).

Dodgen and Brickman state similar goals in their discussion of psychotherapy offered to maladjusted Marine recruits (1967). One possible explanation of the pressures leading to rapid return of the psychologically disturbed to active participation emerges from Coleman's analysis of psychological symptoms in the armed forces. According to Coleman, successful adaptation to military life depends on group cohesion and solidarity; overtly expressed psychological symptoms threaten this solidarity. Coleman describes the problems which such symptoms pose for the group: "The emergence of symptoms as acutely felt experiences is a signal in the patterning of meaningful group experience. It may be regarded as an index of social disorder" (1967:166).

The functions of the sick role for group solidarity are clear: When deviance becomes overt, the sick role isolates the individual temporarily from other soldiers in his unit, thereby protecting their morale and efficiency. Moreover, since an individual who adopts the sick role in the armed forces experiences strong pressures to return to his unit, deviance through the assumption of the sick role does not become widespread.

On the other hand, there are subtle counterpressures which retard the "recovery" of some soldiers. First, as Schneider demonstrates, the peers with whom an individual associates in basic training before he adopts the sick role tend to reject him while he occupies the role. In resuming his responsibilities, an individual must also achieve a new position among his peers, who may have viewed his stay in the hospital, at least in part, as a way of "goofing off." For this reason, some men who adopt the sick role in the armed forces become fixed in it; the longer they are away from their active peers, the harder it is to return (Schneider, 1964:392).

Second, military physicians certify illness and insure adoption of the sick role by certain soldiers whose behavior has created disciplinary problems within their units. In such cases, company commanders enter into a delicate process of negotiation with medical officers to effect separation of the troublesome soldier from his unit on the basis of medical or psychiatric unsuitability. For example, when a soldier's ability or motivation for military service is questioned, especially on the basis of disciplinary infractions, he is referred to a military psychiatrist for evaluation. Daniels analyzes this process:

> . . . company commanders must have the evaluation of the psychiatrist on record before they can initiate a separation request for one of their men. If the psychiatrist recommends a "further trial of duty," the commander will have difficulty in persuading higher channels to honor his request to separate a man. The psychiatrist lends weight to the commander's request for a separation if his evaluation suggests that some kind of mental incapacity is present. The psychiatrist's expertise can be used to justify a separation where otherwise the question of the commander's leadership and judgment in the management of a difficult soldier might have been raised. Such considerations in the situation may be reflected directly in the diagnosis of the case. Thus all parties involved come to understand that the requirement for a psychiatrist's evaluation may affect not only the future career of a difficult soldier but also, on occasion, the career of his commanding officer as well (1969: 260).

When a soldier's behavior causes difficulty for his commanding officer, the military medical system can stretch the criteria for entry into the sick role. In this way the sick role functions as a route by which the armed forces can control deviance and reduce disciplinary problems. Whether or not the soldier returns to active duty, the sick role has served a temporary function for both the individual and the social system (cf. Melville, 1952). It has provided a more-or-less legitimate escape route for the individual, while it has controlled his deviance by removing him temporarily from his unit.

THE MILITARY DRAFT

> GUESTS (resuming conversation . . .):
> ". . . . Anyway, the war's over. It's something they can't draft you any more."
> The dying man sits bolt upright in bed. He listens
> —Bertolt Brecht, **The Caucasian Chalk Circle** (1965:75).

An unpopular war creates widespread opposition to a government in power, especially among those subject to conscription. Draft-eligible men who object to their country's war policy form a potential source of political instability. If a country provided no alternative role for men who wished not to participate in a given war, the possibility of dissension and even revolt—in both military and civilian life—would increase. Therefore a regime must establish carefully controlled mechanisms by which individuals can deviate from military obligations without threatening political stability. In addition to conscientious objection, occupational deferments, and dependency deferments, the sick role provides such a mechanism.

As opposition to the Indochina War has grown in the United States, and as more draftable youths have become unwilling to serve in the armed forces, medical certification of unsuitability for service has become increasingly valued. Physicians in the United States traditionally have served as certifiers of medical suitability; doctor's approval often is required for certain jobs, insurance, admission to certain schools, travel, and other activities. The widespread demand for medical certification of unsuitability, however, seems to be a relatively recent phenomenon in the United States.

To help meet this demand, several organizations have established medical and psychiatric services for draft-eligible men. For example, the Medical Committee for Human Rights (MCHR) has worked with draft counselling agencies in several cities to provide physical examinations for individuals subject to the draft. These services have been offered at nominal charge; if potentially disqualifying conditions are found, letters of certification are sent to the individual's local draft board. Figure 4 shows rates of utilization of these services.

Individuals who cannot claim physical reasons for exemption may present psychiatric evidence of unsuitability. The draft counselling service of the American Friends Service Committee, together with MCHR, has offered a staff of consulting psychiatrists who provide their services to youths who believe they are psychically unfit for service. Partly in response to increased public interest in the grounds of medical exemption, the Department of the Army also has facilitated the certification of medical unsuitability by releasing for public distribution the regulations pertaining to medical standards. Since 1968, the publication *Medical Service— Standards of Medical Fitness* has been available for sale to the general public through the United States Superintendent of Documents (U.S., Department of the Army, 1967).

Have these developments been associated with an increasing rate of medical disqualification over the course of the Indochina War? That is, how successful have young men been in obtaining certification necessary to enter the sick role? Many draft counselling agencies have reported cases of individuals who have vocally enunciated political opposition to the military at their preinduction physical examinations and who subsequently have received medical deferments. Although these political deferments are extremely difficult to document quantitatively, the Department of the Army has published raw data whose analysis indicates that an increasing number of draft-liable men have entered the sick role during the war (U.S., Department of the Army, 1969). Figure 5 demonstrates that medical disqualifications rose steadily between 1965 and 1968. The disqualification rate increased both for individuals who had not been examined previously and for those who had a previous examination (the latter group included mostly individuals who received deferments because of temporarily incapacitating medical conditions and who were reexamined at a later point in time).

Recognizing that over-all medical disqualifications rose over the course

Figure 4. Draft-eligible males examined and advised by Medical Committee for Human Rights, April 1968–Jan. 1970

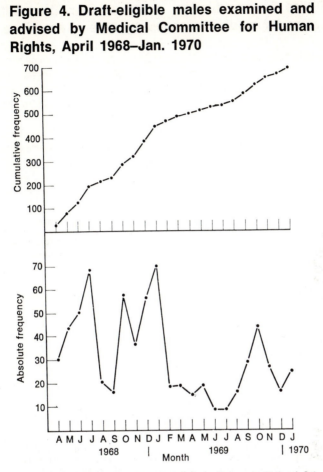

Source: "Latent Functions of the Sick Role in Various Institutional Settings" by Howard Waitzkin, in Social Science and Medicine 5 (1971):61. Reprinted courtesy of Pergamon Press, as taken from Statistical notes (anonymous), Medical Committee for Human Rights, P.O. Box 382, Prudential Station, Boston, Mass., 02199.

Although physical examinations also were provided prior to April 1968, statistical notes for that period are not available. The above data reflect services in the Boston area only; similar programs were operating in Chicago, San Francisco, and other cities.

of the war, one may then ask if different groups in the society had differential access to the sick role. Data to help answer this question are available on the basis of race but not class or other demographic characteristics. As shown in Figure 6, the disqualification rate for medical reasons increased for both white and black men during the war. However, the rate of medical disqualification for whites was higher by about 10 percent than that for blacks during the entire period, and the rate rose slightly

Figure 5. Preinduction examinations: Disqualification for medical reasons, by type of examinee

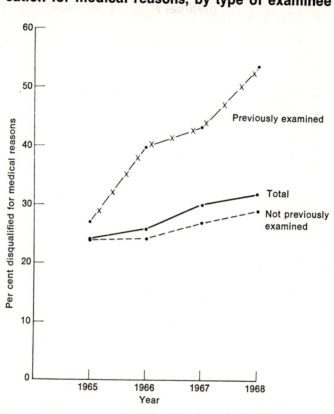

Source: "Latent Functions of the Sick Role in Various Institutional Settings" by Howard Waitzkin, in Social Science and Medicine 5 (1971):62. Reprinted courtesy of Pergamon Press, as taken from U.S., Department of the Army (1969:15).

faster for whites than for blacks (7.8 percent for whites between 1965 and 1968, 5.9 percent for blacks). As indicated by these data, the sick role as an alternative to military service appears to be somewhat more readily accessible to whites than to blacks.

The relationship between disqualifications for medical reasons and those for mental reasons yields further information about differential access to the sick role. As part of preinduction processing, all individuals subject to the draft are administered a battery of psychological tests. This testing is designed as a screening device to assure minimum intellectual capacity for adequate functioning in the military. Under the impact of intensified American efforts in Vietnam, three changes in mental qualifications for induction occurred in 1965 and 1966. The effect of these changes was to lower minimum mental requirements for service, so that

Figure 6. Preinduction examinations: Disqualification for medical reasons, by race

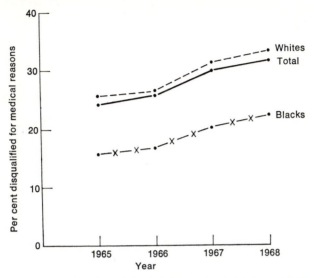

Source: "Latent Functions of the Sick Role in Various Institutional Settings" by Howard Waitzkin, in Social Science and Medicine 5 (1971):63. Reprinted courtesy of Pergamon Press, as taken from U.S., Department of the Army (1969:40).

many individuals who previously had been classified as unqualified on the basis of mental capacity then could be inducted (Karpinos, 1967).

It might be expected that this lowering of mental requirements would have a differential effect on various groups in society; specifically, it would lead to the increased induction of individuals with limited educational opportunities. As illustrated in Figure 7, the over-all percentage of disqualifications for blacks fell markedly as compared to whites immediately after the new mental standards were instituted. Figure 8 shows decreases in percentage of disqualifications for mental reasons, as compared to increases in disqualifications for medical reasons, among whites and blacks between 1965 and 1968. Because of the change in mental requirements, disqualifications for mental reasons decreased much more sharply among blacks than among whites. At the same time medical disqualifications increased for both racial groups, but slightly more so for whites. The percentage decrease in mental disqualifications for whites appeared to be balanced by an increase in medical disqualifications. No such balancing effect occurred among blacks; the percentage decrease in mental disqualifications was much larger than the increase in medical disqualifications. Although whites' access to the sick role appears to have offset the effects of reduced mental requirements, such a mechanism does not seem to have operated for blacks. It appears that black

Figure 7. Preinduction examinations: Disqualification for all reasons, by race

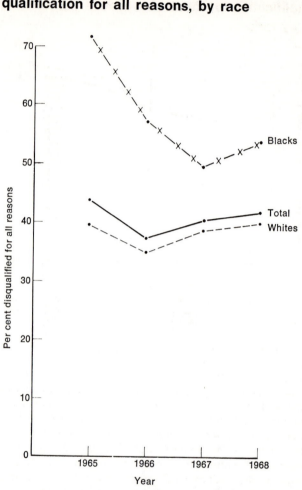

Source: "Latent Functions of the Sick Role in Various Institutional Settings" by Howard Waitzkin, in Social Science and Medicine 5 (1971):64. Reprinted courtesy of Pergamon Press, as taken from U.S., Department of the Army (1961:40).

men with relatively deprived educational backgrounds, previously disqualified for mental reasons, were drafted with increasing frequency. Individuals with stronger educational backgrounds—potential sources of articulate opposition to the military draft—apparently were granted the opportunity to enter the sick role.

The differential availability of the sick role also is illustrated in the disqualification rates for individuals who had been examined previously

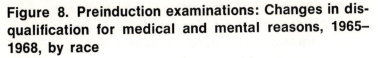

Figure 8. Preinduction examinations: Changes in disqualification for medical and mental reasons, 1965–1968, by race

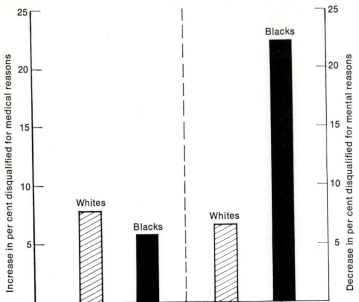

Source: "Latent Functions of the Sick Role in Various Institutional Settings" by Howard Waitzkin, in Social Science and Medicine 5 (1971):65. Reprinted courtesy of Pergamon Press, as taken from U.S., Department of the Army (1969:40).

and presumably had been found temporarily incapacitated at that time. Disqualifications for medical reasons of previously examined individuals increased among both whites and blacks between 1966 and 1968 (Figure 9). Throughout this period, however, medical disqualification at reexamination remained approximately 15 percent lower for blacks than for whites, even though both groups presumably had been found unqualified at previous examination. It appears that blacks who enter the sick role have experienced greater difficulty than whites in retaining the role when they are reexamined.

Whites and blacks have had differential access to the sick role throughout the country, but there also have been regional variations. Figure 10 gives the geographical distribution of draftees inducted into military service in 1968 and shows that three-fifths of all black draftees came from the South. As shown in Figure 11, the medical disqualification rate for Southern blacks was the lowest in the nation, while the rate for Southern whites was comparable to that for whites in other regions. These data indicate that Southern blacks have had less access to the sick role not only than Southern whites but also than black men in other regions of

Figure 9. Preinduction examinations: Disqualification for medical reasons among previously examined individuals, by race

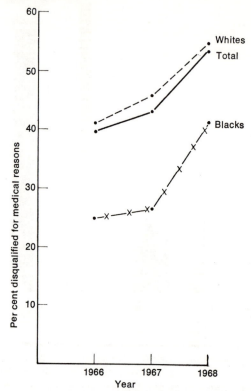

Source: "Latent Functions of the Sick Role in Various Institutional Settings" by Howard Waitzkin, in Social Science and Medicine 5 (1971):65. Reprinted courtesy of Pergamon Press, as taken from U.S., Department of the Army (1969:43).

the country. Moreover, it can be seen that Figures 10 and 11 are nearly mirror images. The contribution of each geographic region and each racial group to the total number of draftees was inversely related to medical disqualifications. For example, while the medical disqualification rate was low and the induction rate high for blacks in the South, both relationships were reversed for blacks in the West. Finally, in Figure 11 the white-black differential in medical disqualifications varied only slightly in different regions. The South showed the largest differential, with 12.7 percent more medical disqualifications among whites than blacks. The differential was smallest in the North Central region, where 8 percent more whites than blacks received medical disqualifications.

Figure 10. Distribution of draftees inducted in 1968, by geographic area and race

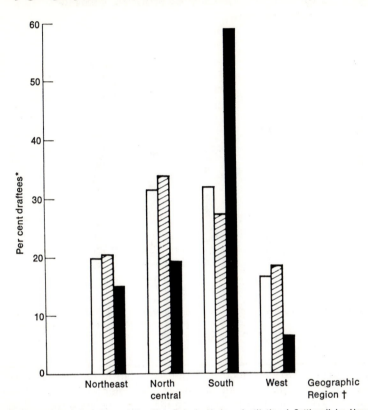

Source: "Latent Functions of the Sick Role in Various Institutional Settings" by Howard Waitzkin, in Social Science and Medicine 5 (1971):66. Reprinted courtesy of Pergamon Press, as taken from U.S., Department of the Army (1969:59).

= Total

= Whites

= Blacks

*Percentages computed on the basis of each group (total, whites, blacks).

†States within each geographic region are as follows: Northeast—Me., N.H., Vt., Mass., R.I., Conn., N.Y., N.J., Pa.; North Central—O., Ind., Ill., Mich., Wis., Minn., Ia., Mo., N.D., S.D., Neb., Kan.; South—Del., Md., D.C., Va., W.Va., N.C., S.C., Ga., Fla., Ken., Ala., Miss., Ark., La., Okla., Tex.; West—Mont., Idaho, Wyo., Col., N.M., Ariz., Utah, Nev., Alaska, Calif., Hawaii, Ore., Wash.

Although military obligations are theoretically universal in American society, many youths for a variety of reasons prefer not to serve. To avoid widespread and disruptive opposition, the society must establish mechanisms by which men can deviate from military obligations within controlled limits. The sick role provides one such mechanism. Especially

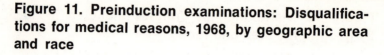

Figure 11. Preinduction examinations: Disqualifications for medical reasons, 1968, by geographic area and race

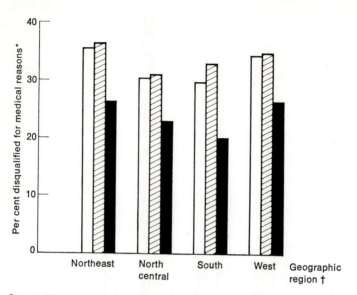

Source: "Latent Functions of the Sick Role in Various Institutional Settings" by Howard Waitzkin, in Social Science and Medicine 5 (1971):67 Reprinted courtesy of Pergamon Press, as taken from U.S., Department of the Army (1969:51).

Key: Same as in Figure 10.

during an unpopular war, access to the sick role is facilitated, although more so for some groups than others. In the Selective Service System, the sick role seems to offer a controlled mode of deviance for individuals who are unable or unwilling to cooperate fully with the system but who will not—once granted medical exemption—actively work to overthrow the system. By expanding access to the sick role (especially for well-educated white men on the East and West Coasts) the Selective Service System has reduced sources of potential opposition within the armed forces.

CONCLUSION: THE SICK ROLE AND SOCIAL CHANGE

We have considered the latent functions of the sick role in a number of institutional settings—the family, the mental hospital, the totalitarian state, the penal institution, the armed forces, and the Selective Service System. In each case, we have emphasized the benefits which the sick role can contribute to the stability of the social system, as well as secondary gain which can accrue to the individual. Because of the inherent methological limitations of functional analysis, we offer these ideas as suggestive rather than conclusive.

There are many other institutions which at times appear to benefit from the sick role. As Szasz has written, physicians associated with university health services—especially psychiatrists—often provide information about students to administrators trying to control disruptions on campus (1967). Absenteeism for illness in some industries may provide a temporary escape from occupational demands which mollifies possible objections to the conditions of work. For example, Weinberg has claimed that upper respiratory infections, which cause an average of seven days of disability per person per year in the United States, are "beneficial since [they] force acceptable periods of rest in an overworked society" (1969). In certain service professions lacking unionization or the right to strike (teachers, nurses, physicians, air traffic controllers, police, etc.), the sick role—when adopted in an organized fashion—offers a convenient tool in bargaining for higher wages. The possible functions of the sick role in these different institutional settings offer a potential for further study.

In conclusion, it is worthwhile to reiterate some of this chapter's implications for institutional change. The role demands which institutions exert frequently come into conflict with the personality needs of individuals. Under these circumstances, institutions face the possibility of dissidence and even rebellion if they do not permit limited deviant behavior. The sick role provides a convenient mechanism of social control by which institutions can allow deviant behavior within carefully controlled limits. Because the sick role reduces potential opposition directed against the institutional structure itself, it fosters institutional stability. From this perspective, the sick role appears to support the institutional status quo. Physicians, often eager to satisfy the personality needs of individual patients, tend to expand their certification of the sick role in such institutional settings as prisons and the Selective Service System. This apparently beneficent act on the physicians' part may result in unintended conservative and perhaps counterrevolutionary consequences, when viewed from the perspective of institutional change.

4 Stratification in Medicine

A person's relation to the means of production is an important, though not the only, determinant of one's class position. Marx attributed primacy to economic production in his analysis of social stratification. In industrial society, capitalists control the means of production; workers, despite their function as producers of goods and services, remain separated from ownership of capital and equipment (1963:122–123). In this distinction, which pertains principally to an individual's position in the economic system, Marx found the origins of stratification and the basis of social class.

MEDICAL CARE AS A DIMENSION OF STRATIFICATION

More recent analysts have noted that stratification transcends economic production alone. People are stratified not only by their roles in production and the wages they earn. Other criteria of stratification are educational background, access to suitable housing, availability of recreational facilities, insurance policies, transportation, and health care (Miller and Roby, 1970). Although these are only a few of the criteria by which a population is stratified, it is clear that they do tend to be clustered. That is, individuals with managerial or professional-level occupations also tend to obtain more advanced educational opportunities, occupy more desirable housing, and so forth. Incongruence among these dimensions of stratification—for example, a highly educated individual who cannot find a high-paying job—is a frequent source of strain (e.g., Lenski, 1956, 1966).

Health care as a dimension of stratification is a much lamented problem, about which capitalist societies have done little. The "two-class system" of medicine in the United States is now widely recognized (cf. Kosa et al., 1969; Waitzkin, 1971). Low-income individuals and families most often have inadequate access to decent health services. Until recent years, people with limited finances who could not afford private fees for services had to rely on charity medicine from the outpatient clinics, wards, and emergency rooms of hospitals. There, care has been fragmented and crisis-oriented, with a frequent turnover of physicians. Alternatively, low-income patients could approach private practitioners and plead poverty, in this case relying on the largesse of physicians to adjust fees according to a "sliding scale." Because the dependability of this approach has been variable, most low-income patients have utilized medical services infrequently, as compared to higher-income groups. Their visits to doctors usually are responses to symptoms which they feel are serious; preventive contacts are rare.

In this way, health care is also clustered with other elements of stratification. Patients who enjoy a high level of income, advanced education, and attractive housing generally have access to superior health care. Preventive physical examinations and other services, as well as efficient responses to medical emergencies, are available to such patients. Despite recent legislation such as Medicare and Medicaid, whose purpose has been to improve services for low-income patients, health care remains maldistributed and inaccessible for much of the population (e.g., Roghmann et al., 1971). Reform measures have not yet eliminated health care as an element of stratification in capitalist society.

STRATIFICATION WITHIN THE MEDICAL SYSTEM

From the perspective of the broader social system, health care is one dimension of stratification. However, within the institution of medicine itself (as defined in Section 1), numerous forms of stratification have evolved which affect the organization of services, relationships among health workers, and the interaction between doctors and patients. There are at least three bases of stratification within medicine: professionalism, elitism, and restricted communication.[3] The first two of these we will discuss briefly, before devoting more detailed attention to the third.

Professionalism As noted previously, stratification no longer derives solely from differential control over the means of production. Increasingly, authority relations in society have become a major source of social hierarchies. As Dahrendorf points out, the "differential distribution of authority invariably becomes the determining factor of systematic social conflicts of a type that is germane to class conflicts in the traditional Marxian sense of this term" (1959:165). Consequently, conflict within a social system develops between groups who hold legitimate authority and those who are subject to this authority.

Perhaps the single most important characteristic of professionalism, especially medical professionalism, is the claim for "autonomy of technique." According to this claim, only highly trained members of the profession possess the expertise needed to evaluate the technical aspects of medicine (Freidson, 1970a:45). Because of this autonomy and exclusive control over one's work, physicians have come to dominate the medical division of labor. Moreover, their authority has broadened to incorporate control over not only the medical, but also the social and economic spheres of health care delivery.

Physicians' authority generally is legitimated on "rational" grounds, to invoke Weber's classic analysis (Weber, 1964:324–429). Thus, it is physicians' technical expertise, rather than their personal charisma or the force of tradition, which enables them to expect acquiescence to their decisions from both patients and subordinate health workers. Beyond the authority of expertise, however, another type of authority has emerged as modern medicine has become more bureaucratized. This is the "authority of office," which accrues to administrators, professors of academic medical specialties, government health officials, and other physicians who occupy superordinate positions within bureaucratic structures (Gouldner,

3. We are by no means suggesting that these are the only sources of stratification within medicine. Others include sexism and racism. While these topics are beyond the scope of this study, they are well documented elsewhere (Boston Women's Health Book Collective, 1973; Ehrenreich and Ehrenreich, 1973).

1954:215–228). Both sources of medical authority, expertise and office, tend to place physicians at the top.

Authority relations in medicine, therefore, have created a stratified health system. Doctors occupy superordinate positions. Patients, on the other hand, hold subordinate positions because of their exclusion from authority within the health system. By virtue of their lack of medical competence, patients have no authority within a technical hierarchy organized around expertise. Furthermore, since their roles as health consumers subsume a subordinate relation to the administrators of medical facilities, patients have essentially no access to authority in the bureaucratic hierarchy. Clearly, then, patients occupy the lowest stratum within the authority structure of the health care system. More specifically, by analogy with Marx's analysis, we suggest that patients might be considered a unique social class.

Since Marx attaches four overlapping meanings to the concept of class, it will be necessary to specify its usage here (cf. Bell, 1972). In the case of the worker, the concept of class includes four usages. First, there is Marx's eschatology whereby civil society will become polarized into two classes: the bourgeoisie who own the means of production, and the proletariat who are excluded from such ownership. The culmination of class conflict between these two groups will be precipitated by the revolutionary action of the proletariat. Through the restructuring of society, communism will be ushered in, and all groups will be reunited in a classless society (Marx and Engels, 1948:30–31).

Secondly, in Marx's analysis, class refers to the structural location of a group of persons in society. Ownership of property, or one's objective relationship to the means of production, is the main criterion for determining the class position of the individual. One's structural position also may be defined more broadly in terms of authority relations within the social system. In this instance, conflict may occur between those classes of persons in authority positions and those whose structural positions deprive them of authority.

Thirdly, classes may be based purely on economic or political interest. Marx applies this concept of class in "The Eighteenth Brumaire of Louis Bonaparte" while explicating the historical role of Napoleon III (Marx and Engels, 1968). Although Napoleon represents no specific class, he successfully manipulates the many political and economic interest groups, qua classes, against each other to take control of the French government. In this usage, the term class refers to each different micropolitical unit which acts on the basis of its own self-interest.

Marx's fourth usage of class concerns class consciousness. He postulates that class consciousness refers to each individual's awareness of structural factors which result in the dehumanization and exploitation, or alienation, of members of his or her class. Only with consciousness of common interests will members of a latent class be ripe for political organization. "On the basis of these class interests, in fighting to realize them or defend them, the groups determined by the distribution of property in production, and by the distribution of political power flowing from it, organize themselves into classes" (Dahrendorf, 1959:15–16). In this instance, political organization around class interests is the criterion for the existence of a class.

By analogy, we suggest that the last three Marxian usages of class can be applied to the situation of patients within medical social structure. As already discussed, health consumers are subordinated to both expert and administrative authority. Consequently, patients share a common structural position within the health system and may be considered a class in the second Marxian sense. The subordination of patients is perpetuated by the concentration of power in the hands of the providers of health care, especially physicians, to the exclusion of health consumers.

As the focus of health care delivery has shifted from the basic doctor-patient relationship to more complex medical institutions, groups other than doctors have begun to participate in the production and distribution of medical services. Insurance companies, drug and medical supply industries, professional associations, health administrators, medical schools, and government are the major units whose political and economic self-interest determine decisions made in the sphere of health care. Health consumers comprise yet another such group, although their influence on health care decision-making has been relatively limited. Thus, Marx's usage of class in the "Eighteenth Brumaire" can be applied to the situation of patients who must compete with other self-interested groups for economic and political power in the health system.

Finally, as a group with latent interests, patients lack class consciousness. If their interests became manifest (Dahrendorf, 1959:179–180), patients would be transformed from a quasi-group to a solidary group—a collection of individuals "who think in terms of the effect of political decisions on the aggregate and feel that they are in some way personally affected by what happens to the aggregate" (Gamson, 1968:19). At this stage, conflicts between the providers and consumers of health care would become a psychological reality to this subordinate group. As a politically organized interest group, patients would be an example of a class in the fourth Marxian sense cited above. The revolutionary potential of such a patient class implies a reorganization of authority relations within medicine to create a health system which no longer oppresses and exploits its consumers.

Furthermore, such a reorganization might alleviate the stratification of health workers which is caused by the dominance of physicians within the medical hierarchy. Nurses, aides, orderlies, ward clerks, and medical social workers (to consider only a few occupational roles within the institution of medicine) generally take orders from above. Despite the widely recognized fact that these subordinate health workers often understand more about patients' total needs and have more extensive daily contact with patients in clinics and hospitals, they generally can contribute little to decisions concerning patient management.

Stratification of health workers, in fact, has become a significant impediment to health care in the United States and in other countries. When decisions about patient care come only from physicians, many human dimensions of medical practice are de-emphasized or overlooked. In this context, it is important to note the attempts of some socialist countries to overcome stratification in medicine.

Cuba has assigned responsibility for public health predominantly to local committees within each community—the Committees to Preserve the Revolution. The principal function of these committees is to work toward the continued political allegiance of the populace to the national communist government. The same committees, however, keep accurate records of health and illness within their locales. They encourage individuals to visit physicians when symptoms arise. In addition, they insure that public health measures, such as immunization programs against communicable disease, are carried out effectively.

Beyond this more active role of non-physicians in health care, Cuban doctors themselves have assumed activities which have brought them closer to other workers. For example, physicians (like other professional or bureaucratic officials) are expected to spend approximately one month per year in harvesting the sugar crop or analogous manual jobs. The purpose of this endeavor is to keep doctors constantly aware of the life experience and needs of working people (Butler, 1969; John et al., 1971; Representatives of Cuban Ministry of Health, 1969; Medical Committee for Human Rights, 1970; Navarro, 1972).

China's attempts to reduce medical stratification have been both more ideological and more practical in scope. During the Cultural Revolution of the late 1960s, hierarchies of all kinds were subjected to severe critical scrutiny and change. In industry, managers were required to assume the role of previously subordinate workers. In medicine, hierarchies involving physicians, nurses, aides, and orderlies were drastically altered. Hospital teams were reorganized so that staff members at all levels made rounds together, discussing therapeutic and management decisions in common. The contribution of aides and orderlies, with less formal training but with a closer feeling for the life situations of most patients, came to be highly respected. More important, a spirit of mutual criticism entered the relationships among staff members. Orderlies and aides became free to criticize the behavior of physicians and nurses who previously had held superordinate positions. Criticisms ranged from comments about aloof and impersonal mannerisms to suggestions about concrete therapeutic decisions (Horn, 1969:53–65). As a result of a wide-ranging ideological attack against the hierarchical structures in Chinese society, the team concept in medicine entered a more meaningful reality.

On a practical level, China has vastly extended the use of paraprofessional health workers in primary patient care. The country has scrupulously avoided the over-training of medical personnel, which in nations like the United States has created reluctance among physicians to practice in rural and some urban areas where advanced technological facilities are unavailable. "Barefoot doctors" are individuals selected by their local communities to attend brief training courses in medicine, lasting from three months to a year. These paraprofessionals then return to their communities, where they continue to spend the majority of their time in their previous agricultural or industrial occupations. However, they also devote a portion of their time to caring for the common illnesses and injuries which arise among people in the communities. Serious or complex problems, which surpass the barefoot doctors' level of competence, are referred to regularly trained physicians who visit rural areas periodically. In acute emergencies, patients are transported rapidly to urban medical centers, where specialists can attend to conditions which demand more advanced training (Horn, 1969:124–183; Sidel, 1972). In this system, the barefoot doctors have obtained a great deal of respect and confidence. They also have been instrumental in overcoming the internal stratification in medicine which inhibits an adequate distribution of health personnel among the populations of many countries.

In both China and Cuba, the redistribution of authority in medicine has also extended to include patients. Local Chinese communities decide who will be sent for training as a barefoot doctor; in hospitals patients contribute to the management of their peers. Similarly, in Cuba laymen are encouraged to participate in health planning for their local communities. Patient interests, therefore, have had an increasing impact on these health systems since the advent of socialism.

Elitism   In most capitalist societies, medical stratification transcends the simple hierarchical structure of occupational roles. Hospitals and medical schools themselves are stratified in terms of economic resources, prestige, and power to control health policy. The emergence of medical imperialism, by which large health organizations seek to expand their clientele and territory, raises many problems which will be discussed in Section 5.

Beyond the issue of medical imperialism, however, lies the much subtler and more difficult issue of elitism. Because of emphasis on the basic sciences, the 1940s and 1950s brought an explosion of technological advances in medicine. Since then, a scientific ideology has held that only a limited number of medical centers can provide top-quality health care. The characteristics of these medical centers are generally quite uniform. They are located in cities, are affiliated with universities, maintain complex facilities for basic science research, and stock technologically advanced equipment which requires large capital investment.

It is difficult to question the need for such medical centers. A limited number of patients will continue to have illnesses complex or severe enough to demand the specialized attention and facilities which only large university-affiliated hospitals can offer. In addition, various diseases remain for which cures may eventually be found through basic science research (though it has been argued that health care in the United States would benefit rather than suffer if all basic research were suspended for a period of years and equivalent funds were made available to distribute present knowledge to a wider segment of the American population).

The prominence of large medical centers in the United States, meanwhile, has led to several distressing effects. Most obviously, they have attracted financial resources and facilities to very limited geographical areas. Those funds which have been available in rural areas—for example, through the Hill-Burton Act—have been spent to construct new hospitals which are frequently underutilized rather than to aid practitioners in attending to more low-income patients, hiring auxiliary paraprofessional workers, sponsoring preventive health programs, and so forth.

Even more striking has been the medical centers' influence on the distribution of physicians. The prestige system of American medicine has encouraged individuals to seek highly specialized training at a relatively small number of elite teaching hospitals. Medical schools often are unabashed in directing medical students toward elite hospitals for internships and residencies. For example, one school has provided the following advice regarding internships to senior students:

> To achieve a balanced list [of hospitals to apply for internship], it is helpful to consider the various hospitals in the three following categories:
> 1. The most coveted
> 2. Those in which a given student's chances are possible
> 3. Those in which his chances are probable (of these, one or two should be almost certain "back-up" appointments)
> Students with top recommendations may with justification list only four or five of the "most coveted" hospitals. Other students, if they are to be matched [i.e., selected by a hospital for internship] must list other hospitals which for them are in the "possible" and "probable" categories. Any student may wish to take a flyer at one or two of the "coveted" hospitals where they [sic] have a chance of being matched. It is, however, pointless for those with a "Satisfactory" [as opposed to "Good" or "Excellent"] recommendation to list the very top hospitals. The bulk of their choices should be in the "possible" and "probable" categories. . . .
> The internship and residency period has been considered by many to be perhaps the most important period of professional education for the physician. It is critical that you work with and learn from the best physicians. Your singular objective should be to obtain the best possible internship available to you. You are urged to select and rank hospitals on the basis of academic merit and without reference to geographical location, work load, duty schedules, and pay scales.
> Although some 80 to 90 hospitals have in the past received applications from [our] students, each year the vast majority of students are matched to the same thirty hospitals (Harvard Medical School, 1971).

The implications of such counselling policies are devastating. First, the most "coveted" hospitals are those which already command an abundance of highly trained physicians. Students are encouraged to strive for internships at these elite medical centers, which consequently have no difficulty in attracting a resident staff. On the other hand, a large number of American hospitals (estimated at 30 to 40 percent) which seek interns and residents annually in approved training programs cannot fill their quotas. Moreover, 43 percent of internships and residencies offered for 1973–1974 could not be filled by the program which matches applicants to available positions (National Internship and Residency Matching Program, 1973; American Medical Association, 1972:21). The "less coveted" hospitals, which are most often located in rural areas or urban ghettoes, thus must remain understaffed or must turn to graduates of foreign medical colleges to provide internship or residency services. Elitism in medicine encourages medical students to obtain postgraduate training, and also to provide health care during this period, in hospitals which usually are already fully staffed with expert physicians; meanwhile, hospitals which desperately need competent house staff must do without.

The implications of elitism extend beyond the internship and residency periods. For many doctors who obtain specialty training in university-affiliated hospitals, these medical centers become umbilical cords. Advanced post-graduate education for physicians results in a "trained incapacity," similar to that Weber described among bureaucratic officials (Weber, 1958a:196–244; Merton, 1968:251–254 et passim). Specialists become accustomed to advanced technological facilities and to patients presenting very challenging diagnostic and therapeutic problems. Upon completion of training, they often feel dissatisfied by the range of relatively commonplace ailments they find in community settings. As a result, they tend to remain closely associated with large medical centers, often advancing slowly along the academic medical hierarchy. Such physicians, who have comprised the dominant trend in American medicine during recent years (Fein, 1967; Fredericks et al., 1971), hesitate to practice in rural or urban areas where their training might remain largely unutilized and where advanced technological facilities are unavailable.

The decision to practice close to academic medical centers frequently is justified on intellectual grounds. On the other hand, specialization itself leads to a relative inability to manage even simple problems outside the sphere of one's specific competence. As a result, the surplus of personnel and facilities near medical centers attracts a further surplus. Cutting the umbilical cord, and practicing in a setting more detached from large teaching hospitals, becomes a fear-evoking experience. Inside academic medical centers, physicians often deride the relatively unsophisticated management of patients with complex problems, who are referred for specialized treatment. Indeed, lack of opportunities for continuing education has created a situation in which the quality of care which local practitioners provide is frequently poor (Lewis and Hassanein, 1970; Peterson et al., 1956). Specialists associated with referral hospitals often view the "local medical doctor" as a technically inferior physician. The true gravity in the situation, however, is that many doctors grow so dependent on large medical centers that they themselves feel inhibited from practicing in areas of great medical need.

Again it is instructive to observe other countries' attempts to overcome elitism in health care. In pre-revolutionary Cuba, for example, Havana's medical school and teaching hospitals contained sophisticated technical facilities and served as the focus of health care for the entire country. Physicians maintained lucrative private practices in Havana and its suburbs; their patients came principally from the professional and entrepreneurial strata as well as the Cuban landed aristocracy. Positions in medical school were difficult to obtain and were available mainly to the children of upper-middle class families. Meanwhile, health care in provincial areas of Cuba remained at the most rudimentary level. Provinces outside Havana did not possess adequate hospitals, let alone medical schools or other teaching facilities. Much of the Cuban peasantry lived their lives deprived of contact with physicians. As a result, morbidity and mortality rates in pre-revolutionary Cuba were among the highest in Latin America.

The immediate response to the revolution by a large part of the Cuban medical profession was emigration. Facing a situation in which private practice concentrated in Havana would be discouraged (in a policy propounded largely by Che Guevara, himself a physician—Guevara, 1968; Harper, 1969), approximately one-third of Cuba's doctors left the country. About one-third to one-half of the emigrants moved to the United States. Although private practice was not banned, its viability dwindled with the popularity of the comprehensive and essentially free care offered by the new national health service. The vast majority of Cuban physicians now work for the Ministry of Public Health. Losses from emigration have been reversed by new doctors recruited from working-class families. Medical education is entirely subsidized by the government; all qualified individuals who desire to enter medicine may do so (size of entering classes is flexible) with tuition paid by federal funds. In return for free medical education, graduates are required to spend two years of practice in Cuba's rural provinces. After that time, they may choose to remain in provincial areas as government-salaried general practitioners, or to return to urban medical centers for specialty training.

In addition to changes in medical education, Cuba has tried to overcome elitism by forming an integrated system of provincial hospitals and medical schools. New medical schools and referral centers have been established in each province. Specialty groups have been decentralized from Havana so that each provincial teaching hospital excels in a given field. As a result, the attractiveness of training or receiving care in Havana has diminished. The more equitable distribution of facilities and services throughout the country has led to a significant improvement in the quality and accessibility of health care in Cuba. Largely because of these changes, recent data on morbidity and mortality show that Cuba has obtained a new position as one of the healthiest nations in Latin America (John et al., 1971).

Professionalism and elitism are two broad problems which contribute to stratification in medicine. But medical stratification arises on a much smaller scale as well—within the doctor-patient relationship itself. One basis of stratification in this more limited sphere is restricted communication. Because communicaton between doctor and patient is a necessary part of health care in all societies, its implications for stratification are perhaps more basic.

RESTRICTED COMMUNICATION AND MEDICAL STRATIFICATION

Stratification and information withholding One person's ignorance is often the basis of another's power. As discussed previously, the "competence gap" between physicians and patients comprises an important source of stratification in medicine. Regardless of patients' educational background in other spheres, their knowledge of pathophysiology and therapy seldom approaches physicians' technical expertise. This discrepancy in knowledge leads to the potential for exploitation. Although Parsons optimistically believes that the competence gap can be bridged by the normative pattern of "trust" (Parsons, 1969:336), other analysts are less sanguine. For example, Freidson emphasizes that doctors' special social position of institutionalized privilege is threatened by the demand that their actions and decisions be explained and justified to laymen: "Insistence on faith constitutes insistence that the client give up his role as an independent adult and, by so neutralizing him, protect the esoteric foundation of the profession's institutionalized authority" (Freidson, 1970b: 143). The physician's ability to control and manipulate information creates a basic asymmetry in the doctor-patient relationship. Professional dominance thus is grounded in a stratified distribution of technical knowledge.

The phenomenon of alienation among patients is also grounded in the manipulation of information. Becoming a patient involves (in Freidson's view) giving up one's role as an independent adult. It also means surrendering the control of one's body to another individual, who presumably understands the interventions and therapies required under a given set of physiological circumstances. In the framework of stratification, there is a certain analogy between the alienation of patients and the alienation of workers in Marx's early analysis. Under capitalism, workers lose control over the means of production and in addition surrender their products to the capitalist. Workers' alienation derives from a process in which the pride of fashioning a completed product is lost, since capitalists own the technical facilities needed for manufacture and derive surplus value from the sales of products which workers make (Marx, 1964:106–119).

Although the analogy is not strict and perhaps is oversimplified, patients become alienated through a similar loss of control, in this case, the control over one's body. In entering the sick role, patients generally are expected to seek technically competent help from a physician with whom they are to co-operate (Parsons, 1951:437). The sick role, therefore, requires patients to surrender their bodies to health professionals in exchange for care. The examination and treatment of the body by a relatively detached physician reduces it to a somewhat impersonal object. The roots of patient alienation lie in this surrender of the body. It may be expected that alienation is exacerbated to the extent that surrender of the body remains a process shrouded in ignorance. Alienation becomes most severe when physicians withhold information about illness and therapy.

Alienation associated with information withholding is a widespread phenomenon in Western medicine. A variety of studies, in both the United States and Great Britain, show that patients tend to be more dissatisfied about the information they receive from their physicians than about any other aspect of medical care (Cartwright, 1964; McGhee, 1961; Duff and Hollingshead, 1968; Skipper and Leonard, 1965; Titmuss, 1963; Frank, 1970). At least in part, the current crisis in American health care is a crisis of confidence, in which patients are becoming increasingly unwilling to tolerate a subordinate position. Not only are consumers now demanding a role in broad health policy; they are also seeking a more knowledgeable and consequently less stratified position within doctor-patient relationships. In recognition of this trend, some groups are advocating the creation of a new paramedical role, that of "physician-friend" or "patient-advocate" or "physician-ombudsman." This individual would act as a mediator between doctor and patient, explaining the details of a patient's illness as well as the diagnostic and therapeutic modalities which the physician recommends. In this way, the problem of fully informed consent would be ameliorated by the intervention of a third, relatively disinterested party.

Patients' uncertainty and physicians' power How does information control support stratification within the doctor-patient relationship? Several sociologists have discussed the uncertainty inherent in medical practice. In his theoretical exposition of the doctor-patient relationship, Parsons points out that uncertainty regarding the outcome of illness increases physicians' frustration (1951:449–450, 466–469). Fox documents the uncertainty experienced by medical students in their education and by both physicians and patients involved in medical research. In addition, she analyzes the frequently nonrational and quasi-magical mechanisms which patients and doctors use to come to terms with uncertainty in the medical sphere (Fox, 1957; 1959; 1970). Although both physician and patient experience uncertainty, the competence gap—which derives from a discrepancy in technical knowledge—means that uncertainty generally is greater for the patient than for the physician.

From a slightly different perspective, several economists have pointed out that uncertainty is one characteristic which distinguishes the medical sector from other sectors of the economy (Arrow, 1963; Fuchs, 1966). Fuchs states, for example, that "very few industries could be named where the consumer is so dependent upon the producer for information concerning the quality of the product." According to Fuchs, consumer ignorance in the health field derives from three causes. First, there is an inherent uncertainty regarding the effect of service on any individual. The lay person cannot know the value of a particular procedure or treatment, especially in cases when the medical profession is far from agreed within itself. Secondly, since medical services are infrequently purchased, consumers tend not to develop expertise about treatment or where to go for it. Thirdly, the medical profession does little to inform consumers. In fact, through restrictions on advertising and price competition, the profession appears to take positive action to keep consumers uninformed (Fuchs, 1966).

Even when doctors are certain about the course of disease or the outcome of therapy, they tend to prolong patients' uncertainty. Davis has found, for example, that physicians delay the communication of prognosis to the families of children with poliomyelitis, long after the physicians have a clear understanding of the children's residual deficits (F. Davis, 1960; 1963). Similarly, as Roth has demonstrated, physicians treating patients with tuberculosis refrain from divulging the expected date of discharge from the hospital (1963). Numerous studies of dying patients have shown that although the vast majority desire to know the facts concerning their condition, most of their physicians (69-90 percent, depending on the study) favor the withholding of information from them (Feifel, 1966; Oken, 1961).

How can one explain the observed tendency of physicians to maintain patients' uncertainty, even when patients prefer to be informed and when the physicians' own uncertainty is reduced? The most obvious answer is based on individual psychology: relating bad news can be an emotionally upsetting experience. Experimental evidence suggests that, as a general phenomenon, individuals hesitate to communicate bad news as opposed to good news (Rosen and Tesser, 1970). Physicians may refrain from such communication more than other groups because of a greater fear of death; several studies have reported a higher fear of death among physicians and medical students than among members of other professions (White, 1969). Such psychological reasons might explain the withholding of information from dying patients or the parents of children with polio, but they do not seem to apply to situations in which information is withheld from patients who are improving over the course of therapy (Roth, 1963).

To explain physicians' inclination to maintain uncertainty in their patients, one can consider a theoretical proposition concerning the source of physicians' power: *physicians' ability to preserve their own power over patients in doctor-patient relationships depends largely on the ability to control patients' uncertainty.* Physicians enhance their power to the extent that they can maintain patients' uncertainty about the course of illness, efficacy of therapy, or specific future actions of the physicians themselves.

This statement is actually an extension of a theory applied in general sociology to the study of bureaucracy. Crozier's comparative studies of bureaucracy have led to the following formulation concerning the relationship between power and uncertainty:

> In such a context, the power of A over B depends on A's ability to predict B's behavior and on the uncertainty of B about A's behavior. As long as the requirements of action create situations of uncertainty, the individuals who have to face them have power over those who are affected by the results of their choice (1964:158).

Using data from observations of supervisor-subordinate relationships, Crozier supports his theoretical proposition that supervisory personnel enhance their own power by maximizing their subordinates' uncertainty regarding the future actions of the supervisors. It should be noted that Crozier employs Dahl's definition of power: "The power of a person A over a person B is the ability of A to obtain that B do something he would not have done otherwise" (Dahl, 1957). However, Crozier's formulation seems equally consistent with Parsons' definition of power as a generalized medium of exchange, which he has used to describe power relationships in several social institutions:

> Hence the power of A over B is, in its legitimized form, the "right" of A, as a decision-making unit involved in collective process, to make decisions which take precedence over those of B, in the interest of the effectiveness of the collective operation as a whole (1966:248).

Incorporating Parsons' definition into Crozier's formulation, one would expect that A's ability to make decisions taking precedence over B depends on A's ability to maintain B's uncertainty regarding A's behavior.

These considerations are readily applicable to the doctor-patient relationship. Just as bureaucratic supervisors enhance their own power by maximizing their subordinates' uncertainty, physicians increase their power by maintaining patients' uncertainty about illness and treatment. This theoretical statement does not imply that the maintenance of uncertainty is intrinsically dysfunctional. As Parsons points out, the physician and patient can be conceptualized as a collectivity, working toward the common goal of therapy (1970). From this viewpoint, physicians' ability to make necessary therapeutic decisions may depend on their power position vis-a-vis that of patients. The less uncertain patients become about the nature of their illnesses and the effects of treatment, the less willing they may be to relinquish decision-making power to physicians. At other times, however, the physicians' maintenance of uncertainty may serve no concrete collective function and may merely satisfy the physicians' psychological need for power. Since physicians probably vary in their need for power, one would expect that this variation among physicians would reflect itself in different tendencies to maintain uncertainty in patients. That is, physicians' need for power, apart from the specific characteristics of particular patients, may affect the way they communicate information regarding illness and therapy.

Others also have commented on the relationship between power and the manipulation of information. In a discussion of the social functions of ignorance, Moore and Tumin point out that ignorance on the part of the consumer of specialized services helps to preserve the privileged position of the dispenser of the services. The implication here is that ". . . the specialist's position may be endangered by 'the patient's becoming his own physician'" (Moore and Tumin, 1949:789). In a report of participant observation in tuberculosis hospitals, Roth states that the more closely a patient's experience and knowledge approach that of a physician, the greater becomes the patient's resistance to giving up control of the service to the physician (1963). In this way, reduced uncertainty of tuberculosis patients concerning the course of their illness appears to diminish the power of physicians within the doctor-patient relationship.

The postulated association between uncertainty and power may help explain physicans' reluctance to reveal information to dying patients. A physician's disclosure of fatal illness is equivalent to a declaration of powerlessness: what need has a dying patient for a physician? Perhaps the patient may rely on a physician for palliative therapy or for supportive concern, but the physician's technical ability to cure has vanished, and admission of this fact implies loss of power. Glaser and Strauss describe a unique situation in cancer wards of a Veterans Administration hospital, where patients are poor and possess no alternative to the free care they receive at the hospital. In contrast to the usual reluctance of physicians to inform cancer patients about their illness (Feifel, 1966; Oken, 1961), physicians on these particular wards do not hesitate to disclose terminality to patients directly. Glaser and Strauss comment, "Since the captive lower class patients cannot effectively threaten the hospital or the doctors, the rule at this hospial is to disclose terminality regardless of the patient's expected reaction" (1965:122). Thus, when the physicians' power is assured because of patients' low socioeconomic status, the control of uncertainty becomes less crucial.

Finally, information itself yields power. In the quite different contexts of both psychological and information theory, Maslow (1963) and Cherry (1966) point out that information allows the recipient to select his own future action from a wider range of possible alternatives. Maslow puts the matter succinctly, "What you *don't* know has power over you; knowing it brings it under your control, and makes it subject to your choice. Ignorance makes real choice impossible" (1963:116).

Uncertainty, though an inherent feature of medical practice, is experienced to a greater extent by patients than by physicians. Information transmitted from physician to patient, by reducing the patient's uncertainty, thus tends to reduce the physician's power within the doctor-patient relationship.

Sociolinguistics and the diffidence of the sick poor Information control reinforces stratification in doctor-patient relationships generally, but especially when significant social-class differences between doctors and patients already exist. Many commentators have considered the special communication problems which arise between upper-class or upper middle-class physicians and working-class patients. One theoretical perspective which is pertinent to these problems is that of sociolinguistics—the study of the relationships between language and social structure.

Numerous studies have demonstrated that working-class patients tend to be diffident in questioning their physicians about illness. Interviewing patients recently discharged from hospitals, Cartwright found that professional and nonmanual workers obtained most of their information about illness by asking their physicians and nurses direct questions. In contrast, the information which partly skilled and unskilled workers received resulted from a passive process in which they were given information without asking; they also tended to receive less information (Cartwright, 1964). Using direct observations of doctor-patient interaction rather than questionnaires, Pratt and co-workers discovered a similar diffidence among low-income patients at a medical clinic:

> What was observed, however, is that the patients in our sample participated with the physicians at an extremely low level. They seldom requested information from the physician (one-third of the patients never asked a single question on any visit), they seldom requested the physician to do anything, and seldom even made a statement to direct the physician's attention to something (1957:223).

Likewise, Korsch and associates, using a combination of observational and questionnaire methods, discovered that parents of children attending a pediatric outpatient facility usually did not state to their physicians what information they expected to find out. Also, only 29 percent of the parents' main worries were expressed to the physician during the medical visit (Korsch et al., 1968; Korsch and Negrete, 1972).

Cartwright attributes the diffidence of working-class patients to four causes: (1) their sense that doctors do not expect them to ask questions; (2) a problem of language which results from patients' ignorance of technical terms which physicians use; (3) the awe with which they regard physicians; and (4) the social distance between patients and doctors, deriving from the doctors' higher class positions. Despite their reluctance to request information, working-class patients differ little from upper-class patients in their desire for information. Although slightly more patients with professional as compared to unskilled occupations want to know the full technical details regarding their illness, there is no general class difference in patients' desire for as much information as possible presented in nontechnical language (Cartwright, 1964).

Moreover, the majority of all hospitalized patients believe that a "good explanation" of illness constitutes one of the most important qualities of a "good doctor" (Skipper and Leonard, 1965). Although they supply no data concerning social-class differences among patients, Reader and co-workers hypothesize that the diffidence of clinic patients may reflect their more generally passive attitude regarding medical care, compared to private patients of higher socioeconomic level. The latter tend to obtain information actively through direct questioning (Reader et al., 1957). The commonly expressed assumption that low-income patients do not want a full explanation of illness seems to be inferred from their hesitation in asking questions, rather than from an actual disinterest in information.

The behavior of working-class patients may be viewed not as an isolated finding, but as a reflection of a more general social-class difference in language use. Knowledge about illness is differentially distributed among members of different social classes. More important, recent theory and research in sociolinguistics indicate that learned linguistic skills appropriate for speaking about illness also may have a differential distribution among classes. Such a distribution of linguistic skills is not a universal feature of societies. For example, in some primitive societies knowledge of disease concepts and names tends to be uniformly distributed among individuals. Since people in these societies are continually exposed to discussions of illness, diagnostic categories are not esoteric subjects, and even children can make fine distinctions among specific diseases (Frake, 1961). In modern societies the possession of linguistic skills pertaining to illness is not uniform and appears to be associated with more general social-class variations in the use of language.

Bernstein's theory and research, together with Lawton's more recent contributions, have elucidated the social-class differences in linguistic skills (Bernstein, 1961, 1962a, 1962b, 1964a, 1964b; Lawton, 1968). Bernstein distinguishes two basic linguistic codes—elaborated and restricted codes—and claims that they are used to a different degree by working-class and middle-class individuals. The principal criterion upon which Bernstein distinguishes the two codes is *predictability:*

> *If it is difficult to predict the syntactic options or alternatives a speaker uses to organize his meanings over a representative range of speech, this system of speech will be called an elaborated code. In the case of an elaborated code, the speaker will select from a wide range of syntactic alternatives and so it will not be easy to make an accurate assessment of the organizing elements he uses at any one time. However, with a restricted code, the range of alternatives, syntactic alternatives, is considerably reduced and so it is much more likely that prediction is possible. In the case of a restricted code, the vocabulary will be drawn from a narrow range but because the vocabulary is drawn from a narrow range, this in itself is no indication that the code is a restricted one (1964a:57).*

In addition to the criterion of predictability, one further distinguishing characteristic is the *expression of intent.* According to Bernstein, in a restricted code, nonverbal rather than verbal signals become the important bearers of changes in meaning. The restricted code "is a facility for the transmission of global, concrete, descriptive, narrative statements in which discrete intent is unlikely to be raised to the level of elaboration and so made explicit" (Bernstein, 1964a:62). Bernstein and Lawton present empirical evidence showing a greater use of an elaborated code by middle-class subjects and a restricted code by working-class subjects.

This sociolinguistic distinction between restricted and elaborated codes helps clarify the observed diffidence of working-class patients within the doctor-patient relationship. Although both working- and middle-class patients want information about their illness, working-class patients do not take as active a role as middle-class patients in asking questions of their physicians. Physicians, using an elaborated code, expect that intent will be expressed verbally and therefore do not provide information, while working-class patients want but do not ask for information through verbal requests. Working-class patients, since they are accustomed to express intent through nonverbal signals, do not state their desire for information verbally. The difference in linguistic codes of physicians and working-class patients thus may lead to a hiatus in communication, because physicians do not become aware of patients' actual communicative intentions. As a result, doctors tend to provide less information than patients expect to receive. Although Bernstein himself has commented on problems of psychotherapy with working-class patients which derive from the utilization of different codes by therapist and patient (1964b), the same problems also seem to apply to communication in general medical practice.

It should also be noted that a person's use of a linguistic code is, to use Chomsky's terms, a question of *performance* rather than *competence.* According to Chomsky, performance denotes the use of language in concrete situations, while competence refers to the speaker's or hearer's actual knowledge of language (1965). Since it is generally assumed that working-class patients lack the capability, or competence, to understand more than the most elementary explanation of disease processes, physicians tend not to talk with them about their illnesses. Physicians' attribution of lack of competence to such patients may derive from a lack of abstraction in these patients' speech. Indeed, Lawton's research has shown that a higher level of abstraction characterizes the elaborated code as opposed to the restricted code. Lawton also has demonstrated that the principal difference between working- and middle-class linguistic patterns involves performance rather than competence. In Lawton's research, working-class boys were capable of using an elaborated code and of enunciating abstractions when required to do so by the investigator's instructions. He concludes that the principal reasons working-class subjects do not use an elaborated code more regularly are lack of practice and, consequently, lack of facility (Lawton, 1968). The implication for medical practice is that working-class patients are capable of understanding information transmitted as part of an elaborated code but that their customary use of a restricted code conveys a false sense of linguistic liability. As a result, physicians fail to convey the information these patients desire and are able to process.

Clinical considerations Beyond the issue of stratification per se, the transmission of information from physician to patient affects both the quality of care and the course of treatment, especially as perceived by the patient. Gaps in the informative process produce defects in clinical practice which will not be corrected by organizational changes in the delivery of care. The communication of information about illness affects patient care in several ways: by enhancing the accuracy of history-taking, by providing more useful medical records, by increasing patients' compliance with therapeutic regimens, by heightening patients' satisfaction, and by improving patients' physiologic and psychologic responses to therapy.

Perhaps the single most important activity in clinical medicine is effective *history-taking.* Patients' ability to provide a meaningful history depends largely on their understanding of prior experience with illness. One of the most common problems in taking a history from new patients derives from their confusion about previous episodes of illness and medical treatment. Part of this confusion results from the patients' imperfect memory or comprehension. However, previous information from the doctor that is incomplete, erroneous, or contradictory also limits the accuracy of a history at a later point in time. The physician's success in transmitting information about illness therefore "feeds back" to a physician through patients' later ability or inability to provide a meaningful history (Figure 12). Although the relationship between lay knowledge and history-

Figure 12. Schematic feedback model of information transmittal and history-taking

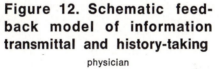

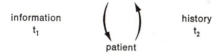

Source: "The Communication of Information about Illness" by Howard Waitzkin and J. D. Stoeckle, in Advances in Psychosomatic Medicine 8 (1972:183). Reprinted courtesy of S. Karger.

t_1 = first point in time.
t_2 = second point in time.

taking has not been studied systematically, it is thought that more detailed information about illness, if supplied to the patient with accuracy and consistency, would reduce the number of serious errors which occur in clinical practice (Medical Defence Union and Royal College of Nursing, 1961). To help improve the quality of transmitted information, a manual of explanations about illness for patients has been prepared (Griffiths, 1968).

In addition to its importance in history-taking, information transmitted to patients also is related to the nature of *medical records.* For the most part, a patient's medical record only contains a description of clinical observations and therapeutic measures. It seldom contains statements about information transmitted to patients during their visits. Because the record provides no details about the informative process, the doctor or perhaps several doctors treating a patient may forget previous explanations between visits and offer contradictory information when the patient next appears. The problem of consistent information is particularly acute in hospitals, where several staff members care for the same patient with no written record of what information each staff member is conveying. The resulting confusion and dissatisfaction among patients has led to the suggestion that a note on patient education be included in the medical record each time the patient is seen (Weed, 1969: 50–52).

Physicians recognize that the success of treatment usually depends on patients' *compliance* with instructions they receive. Several studies have shown that compliance is closely related to the quality of information which the physician provides. For example, a negative correlation has been found between compliance and "non-reciprocal informativeness," the latter variable derived from a factor analysis of tape-recorded doctor-patient interaction. That is, when doctors provide disproportionately little information as compared to that supplied by patients, the patients tend to comply less with their doctors' orders (M. Davis, 1968). The compliance of mothers in following medical advice concerning their children depends on the extent to which a physician fulfills their expectations of information and provides a detailed explanation about the children's illness (Francis et al., 1969). In addition, knowledge about diabetes in adult patients, presumably deriving from a physician's explanations, is positively correlated with the patients' satisfactory performance of therapeutic recommendations (Williams et al., 1967). Through these effects on patient compliance, the quality of information transmitted from physician to patient influences the efficacy of therapy in clinical medicine.

Patient satisfaction is another goal toward which physicians aim in clinical practice. The dissatisfaction of patients, when it occurs, is most often tied to insufficient, contradictory, or confusing information. This finding has been observed in many studies of hospitalized patients (Cartwright, 1964; McGhee, 1961; Duff and Hollingshead, 1968; Skipper and Leonard, 1965; Titmuss, 1963; Frank, 1970). Moreover, in pediatric practice, dissatisfaction among parents is greatest in those who expect to learn the causation and nature of their child's illness but whose expectations are not met (Korsch et al., 1968). These findings indicate that patient satisfaction is dependent, at least in part, on the information a physician chooses to communicate.

Finally, there is a growing body of evidence which demonstrates a relationship between the transmittal of information and *physiologic and psychologic changes* in patients during hospitalization, especially for surgical procedures. Studies show that postoperative psychological disturbances are minimized if patients receive preoperative information which conveys a concrete picture of what they will perceive after surgery. Such communication permits the patient to accomplish the "work of worrying," which is considered a prerequisite for adequate postoperative adjustment. Absence of preoperative fear, and the consequent occurrence of postoperative psychological disturbance, is largely attributed to a lack of information about the impending stresses of surgery (Janis, 1958). When patients receive detailed information from an anesthetist in the immediate preoperative and postoperative periods, it is found that the postoperative analgesic requirement for narcotics is reduced by approximately one-half. Thus the experience of pain following surgery is mitigated by the structured transmission of information from physician to patient (Egbert et al., 1964). Such salutory effects of information also can be mediated through family relations. Among children whose mothers received detailed information about surgery from a special nurse, several physiological measures (blood pressure, heart rate, postoperative emesis, voiding, and fluid consumption) indicated a more satisfactory recovery from tonsillectomy. These findings support the hypothesis that children's stress in surgery can be relieved by the transmittal of information to mothers; the latter informative process reduces stress in the mothers and indirectly leads to physiological improvements in the children themselves (Skipper and Leonard, 1968).

On "the pedagogy of the oppressed." Just as medical stratification depends in part on patients' ignorance, revolutionary change in the health system requires changes in information transmittal. The process by which patients receive frank, detailed, and humanistically oriented information is essentially an educational process. Its revolutionary potential resembles that which Freire discusses in the context of education in the Third World:

> *Problem-posing education, as a humanist and liberating praxis, posits as fundamental that men subjected to domination must fight for their emancipation. . . . Problem-posing education does not and cannot serve the interests of the oppressor. No oppressive order could permit the oppressed to begin to question: Why? . . . .*
> *We can legitimately say that in the process of oppression someone oppresses someone else; we cannot say that in the process of revolution someone liberates someone else, nor yet that someone liberates himself, but rather that men in communion liberate each other (1970:74, 128).*

In medicine, the "pedagogy of the oppressed" (to invoke Freire's term) would involve an attempt to reduce information withholding and to provide patients with adequate knowledge of diagnosis and therapy. Moreover, it would mean that health consumers could rationally organize themselves into groups which could make meaningful policy decisions for new health programs. "Consumer participation" in health planning will remain largely a matter of co-optation until patients are able to acquire sufficient knowledge about medical care. Otherwise, professionals can continue to propound the notion that only doctors, because they possess special technical skills, can function as the arbiters of health policy.

It is interesting to note that socialist countries which have tried to overcome stratification in medicine have also attempted to increase the amount of information provided to patients. For example, in the People's Republic of China, norms have evolved which encourage physicians to communicate fully with patients about diagnosis, therapy, and prognosis. The withholding of information has become extremely rare, and most patients are fully informed about their conditions. In fact, in many hospitals patients have become active members of ward teams, accompanying doctors and nurses on rounds, serving as intermediaries between health workers and severely ill patients, and commenting on the personal attention which patients are receiving (Horn, 1969). A well-informed patient population has been the logical concomitant of the broad sociopolitical changes occurring in China. Patient education has contributed significantly to de-stratification in the health system.

Stratification in medicine is grounded in the class structure of a society. As we have seen, medical care is one dimension of social stratification. In addition, stratification *within* the institution of medicine is tied to professionalism, elitism, and restricted communication. Overcoming medical stratification will ultimately depend on broader sociopolitical changes in society, whose ramifications will make themselves felt in many other institutions besides medicine.

5   On Medical Imperialism

Men build empires on others' shoulders. In Lenin's classic analysis of imperialism, it was the shoulders of the working class which supported the imperialist ventures of international capitalism (1939). Empire building, however, occurs at many levels; imperialism by nation states is only one (though perhaps the most widely studied) example. Nations extend hegemony over other nations, it is true. But within nations, empire building also takes place at the institutional level and even in interpersonal relations. As many critics have pointed out, medical imperialism lies near the heart of the current health crisis in the United States (Health Policy Advisory Center, 1970; Bodenheimer et al., 1972).

Because medical imperialism is a multifaceted phenomenon, it is difficult to define. In general, it comprises the attempt of large health organizations (medical schools, hospitals, the insurance industry, companies manufacturing medical equipment, and so forth) to expand their physical plants, services, programs, patient populations, or sales. Empire building in medicine, as in other social institutions, occurs at both the organizational and individual levels. For example, medical schools may attempt to add new buildings to their physical plants by buying adjacent property in urban areas, destroying existing houses, and constructing additional facilities. Alternatively, hospitals may sponsor new programs which are based on advanced technology (such as radiation therapy or transplantation units) or which extend health services to nearby communities (such as the sponsorship of health maintenance organizations). By expanding physical plants or starting programs, these organizations enhance their financial resources, power, and prestige. Beyond these examples of organizational imperialism, empire building occurs *within* organizations—for instance, the frequently observed attempt by professors or other faculty members to increase their laboratory space in medical centers.

Medical imperialism leads to many detrimental effects. Some of these effects pertain to the cost and distribution of health care itself. Empire building inevitably produces overlap and duplication. As a result, in many cities one finds a multiplicity of technologically advanced facilities, which often compete with each other for patients. Each hospital feels a need for its own unique transplantation team, coronary-care unit, or other major facility. The prestige of a hospital often is seen to depend on the development of such programs, all of which involve heavy capital expenditures. Coordination through comprehensive planning on a regional basis is a widely discussed but rarely implemented goal (Bodenheimer, 1969; Komaroff, 1971). Because of duplication and overlap, health costs rise, while appropriate facilities remain poorly distributed outside metropolitan medical centers. Furthermore, within urban areas, duplicated facilities often remain under-utilized.

Other detrimental effects of medical imperialism relate not to health care per se, but to the many human needs of people who live near urban medical centers. Increasingly, medical schools and hospitals in cities are experiencing pressures to expand but find that empty land suitable for new buildings is unavailable. Under these circumstances, the tendency of medical centers has been to acquire nearby residential property and gradually to displace the predominantly low-income occupants. While creating the opportunity to expand the centers' physical plants, the acquisition of urban residential property has enabled medical centers to destroy low-income housing. In such instances, medical centers' expansionary policies often conflict with the housing needs of low-income urban residents (cf. Waitzkin, 1970; Duhl, 1969; Health-PAC Bulletin, 1972:24).

The motivations of empire building in medicine are complex. Emphasizing the economic bases of imperialism, Lenin focused on the interest of large cartels and banks in the development of colonial markets and sources of raw materials. By analogy from the Leninist perspective, one expects to find significant economic motivation in the expansion of large medical institutions. Indeed, as discussed later, financial considerations are important in the current enthusiasm of medical schools, hospitals, and the insurance industry for national health insurance and health maintenance organizations.

However, as Weber recognized, stratification transcends mere financial privilege; its bases also include prestige and power (1958b). Medical organizations are stratified in terms of prestige and power, as well as financial position. Issues of prestige influence many imperialist decisions in medicine. When technological hardware is highly valued, for example, it is difficult for hospitals to resist the temptation to build new radiation therapy units, to assemble transplant or cardiac surgery teams, and so forth—even though these efforts may duplicate those of other nearby hospitals. Similarly, by expanding the population served by a large medical center, administrators enhance their own power over new programs, personnel, and patient options. Increased power from new health facilities provides another important motivation for medical imperialism.

Beyond considerations of finances, prestige, and power are certain basic expansionary tendencies which inhere in all large organizations. Banfield has referred to these tendencies as "maintenance and enhancement needs" (1961). According to Banfield's analysis, organizations search for new programs or projects to insure continued viability. In this view there is a logic in organizational activities which transcends concrete issues of finances, prestige, and power—though all three of these classic elements of stratification also influence organizational behavior. By the logic of maintenance and enhancement needs, officials look for novel ways to develop programs, construct facilities, and carry out other expansionary maneuvers. To justify its continued existence, to attract outside support, and to preserve internal morale, an organization must provide evidence that it is *building* rather than remaining at a steady level of performance—the latter being viewed as akin to stagnation. Because all organizations experience maintenance and enhancement needs, the potential for empire building is always present.

Medical organizations differ from others, however, because of the persuasiveness of the ideology which medical men propound. It is difficult to argue with physicians that new hospitals, health research units, or other facilities are not needed, even when this conclusion is obvious. Although planning for expansion rarely takes into account the comprehensive needs and resources of whole communities, saying no to new health projects is hard to do. Even when little justification for expansion can be formulated, its proponents tend to invoke ideological lines which are difficult to resist. First, new facilities are needed to treat sick patients, or to find cures for fatal diseases, or to increase the health resources available to a community. This is the *helping* ideology, which contains elements of *noblesse oblige* strikingly reminiscent of the ideological line enunciated by international colonialists (Fanon, 1967). Much as territorial expansion was needed to bring civilization to indigenous populations, the helping ideology allows medical men to claim that new facilities are required to deliver better health care to the sick.

Decisions about expansion usually do not derive from realistic appraisal of resources and needs by objective observers outside the profession. When outside appraisal is brought to bear, much (if not most) medical expansion is found to be unnecessary (Massachusetts Department of Public Health, 1972; California Department of Public Health, 1972:94–128, 385–398). Usually, however, medical men feel that only they can make such decisions. As a premise, they invoke a second ideological line, that of *medical expertise.* Only doctors or other trained professionals, it is claimed, possess the technical knowledge to make rational decisions about what new facilities are needed. This ideology contains the seeds of empire building. As Freidson puts it, "The [medical] worker . . . develops around it [his work] an imperialism that stresses the technical superiority of his work and his capacity to perform it" (1970b:160). Yet, as discussed in Section 2, professional autonomy has contributed in fundamental ways to the present crisis in health care. Controlling the imperialism of medical expansion will go hand in hand with controlling professional autonomy.

The following discussion is an analysis of recent trends in American health care delivery. As examples of medical imperialism and the exploitation of illness, these trends serve to maintain and enhance large health organizations. Our purpose is not to condemn the individuals who administer these organizations, who often are genuinely concerned about improving the quality and availability of health care. Rather it is to set forth some mechanisms by which organizational interests lead to medical imperialism—which results in fragmented health services and patient populations more often exploited than adequately served.

HEALTH MAINTENANCE ORGANIZATIONS AND NATIONAL HEALTH INSURANCE: WHO WILL BENEFIT?

Among its many troubles, the United States now faces a crisis in health care. This crisis has become particularly salient within the last few years as public opinion has come to bear on the soaring costs of medical services. However, cost is only one of several aspects of the current medical crisis. The others include maldistribution of health services regionally as well as among different socioeconomic strata of American society; the resulting poor quality of medical care in this country, given the trained personnel and technological resources available; and the concentration of power in the hands of the providers of health care rather than health consumers.

Skyrocketing medical costs have been especially problematic since the passage of Medicare and Medicaid. Since 1965 health costs have increased 11 to 12 percent per year, in contrast to 7 to 8 percent per year for the previous 15 years. Public spending is increasing more quickly than private spending: a 15 percent public rate as opposed to a 10 percent private rate increase per year (Rice and Cooper, 1970). Large medical centers benefit from the growth in public spending since an increasing proportion of their expenses are underwritten by these funds. Public funding contributes to medical imperialism by permitting medical centers to develop special programs, purchase equipment, construct new facilities, and so forth, with the assurance that the major portion of the ensuing costs will be paid.

Ironically, patients themselves frequently do not benefit from public health expenditures. For much of the population, health care is becoming financially prohibitive. A major extended illness at contemporary costs can cause bankruptcy for an average American family (Fortune Magazine, 1970). Rising medical costs exacerbate the inequitable distribution of health care within the population. Huge numbers of Americans are simply too poor to afford proper care. In acute situations, these persons are forced to depend on hospital outpatient departments and emergency rooms. For less pressing problems they simply do without appropriate care, since they cannot afford to pay for it.

As discussed earlier, "vertical" maldistribution, based on income, is accompanied by "horizontal" maldistribution of health services, based on geographic disparities in health services. The majority of available physicians and facilities are concentrated in a small number of urban areas, so that many rural districts and low-income areas of cities are medically neglected. Urban medical centers have contributed to this problem insofar as their priorities stress empire building over patient care. Medical schools and related hospitals have shown more interest in research than in direct services to patients. Because young physicians have become overspecialized, their interest in patient care has waned. Consequently, they have gravitated toward prestigious academic institutions, thereby enhancing the maldistribution of services (Fein, 1967). They have lost interest in the commonplace ailments of general practice, where their elaborate training, they feel, would be wasted.

Clearly, medical care is financially or geographically inaccessible to many Americans. The United States' basic health statistics show that huge health care expenditures have had limited impact. In 1971 the United States ranked twenty-fifth in infant mortality and was exceeded by approximately twenty-two other nations in life expectancy at birth (United Nations, 1972a:76–80, 1972b:746–765). American health care delivery is functioning at less than an optimal level, given available resources.

Health providers maintain their power in health care by functioning cooperatively. Six types of organizations—the professional associations, medical schools, hospitals, insurance companies, medical supply industries, and governmental agencies—are highly integrated through a variety of financial, legal-political, and personal links (Lasker, 1971). Commonality of interest among these organizations is enhanced by specific relationships among groups or individuals.

First, a personnel exchange relationship exists whereby individuals who have a major decision-making role in one organization are also influential in another organization. For example, a person connected with health insurance who is made chairman of the presidential task force to study medical care—as in the case of Walter T. McNerney, president of Blue Cross (Health-PAC Bulletin, 1969:6)—creates a convergence of interests between the task force and the insurance industry. Similarly, medical schools are linked to private industry in this manner; business executives are often on the schools' boards of trustees. Corporations producing medical supplies exchange trustees and staff with hospitals, as well as providing consultants to each other and to government planning agencies. Likewise, doctors sit on the boards of insurance, pharmaceutical, and medical supply companies.

A second type of relationship pertains to legal obligations or privileges through either contracts or powers of legitimation. Hospitals are linked to professional associations in this type of relationship since they depend on the Joint Commission on Accreditation of Hospitals—formed by the American Medical Association, the American Hospital Association, the American College of Physicians, and the American College of Surgeons in 1952—for accreditation (Hapgood, 1969; Somers and Somers, 1967). This is one example of the more general need on the part of health personnel, hospitals, and the health industry to be legitimated by the dominant medical profession.

Finally, organizations or individuals may be linked through a convergence of major financial interest or a relationship of direct ownership. The American Medical Association (AMA) depends heavily on income from advertising in its journal, particularly by drug companies. Such advertising is also to the advantage of the pharmaceutical companies, since approximately two-thirds of practicing physicians rely on the advice of the drug industry in deciding what to prescribe for their patients (Greenberg, 1965:281). This reciprocal relationship results in an interlocking of AMA and drug industry interests. Similarly, hospitals depend on insurance companies for patients' payments. Thus, when insurance companies propose an increase in their premiums, they are supported by voluntary hospitals (The Financing Workshop, 1969:4–6). Again mutual interests, especially in the medical economic sphere, result in cooperative exchanges among the providers of health care.

Many of the links among different health organizations consist of a combination of these types of relationships. The ensuing "medical-industrial complex" and its continued expansion have contributed greatly to the health care crisis.[4]

Proposals for solutions to the health crisis center on two innovations: national health insurance (NHI) and health maintenance organizations (HMOs). It is especially important to evaluate these innovations critically within the context of medical imperialism. Although many variations of these ideas have emerged, they can be summarized simply.

National health insurance   NHI is a method of *financing* medical care. Under NHI, the federal government would insure payment for health services. Low-income patients presumably would not face prohibitive

4. Although a detailed economic analysis of the medical-industrial complex is beyond the scope of this section, its financial structure resembles that of "monopoly capital" in other sections of the economy (cf. Baran and Sweezy, 1966; Kelman, 1971).

financial barriers in seeking care. NHI would be administered by the present insurance industry, which would receive government subsidies for low-income patients, or by an independent federal bureaucracy.

Health maintenance organizations In addition to NHI, HMOs figure prominently in current health planning. An HMO is a group of physicians and other health personnel who organize themselves into a working unit, often serving a specific population of patients. Many (but not all) HMOs receive fees on a prepaid basis; in this case the HMO may be referred to as a prepaid group practice. Patients who obtain medical care from a prepaid practice generally pay an annual "capitation" fee, which covers all services and hospitalization they may require. Most plans for NHI include provisions supporting HMOs. HMOs, funded by capitation payments from the federal government, comprise a basic part of the Nixon Administration's proposals for improved health care (U.S., House of Representatives, 1971). Various other plans for NHI, such as that sponsored by Senator Edward Kennedy and Representative Martha Griffiths, encourage the establishment of HMOs by providing special financial incentives (Olson, 1971).

Following the prototypes of the Kaiser-Permanente system in California and the Health Insurance Plan of New York, a number of medical schools recently have become sponsors of HMOs. In several cases, commercial insurance companies and Blue Cross have assumed active roles by underwriting portions of the risks incurred by these HMOs or by offering their subscribers the option of joining HMOs.

Spokesmen for the combination of NHI and HMOs commonly cite three major goals which they hope to attain: improving distribution of health services, reducing costs of health care, and enhancing quality of medical care (Kennedy, 1971: Sections 47, 87, 103; Kennedy, 1972; Perrott and Chase, 1969; Weinerman, 1968; Greenberg and Rodburg, 1971). We contend that these service goals mask many of the real issues involved in the current interest in NHI and HMOs.

We suggest, instead, that these manifest goals diverge greatly from the latent goals of NHI-HMO proposals. Manifest goals refer to goals which are made public and are acknowledged by all participants of the system. Latent goals, on the other hand, are those unspoken goals of the various groups which advocate a particular plan or program. Before evaluating the attainability of the manifest goals of NHI-HMO proposals, we need to examine the latent goals, especially in terms of their implications for medical imperialism.

Specifically, three major types of organizations stand to reap great advantages from NHI and HMOs: medical schools and their teaching hospitals, the present insurance industry, and professional associations. Furthermore, private profit-making corporations not directly involved in the health industry may gain as well. NHI and HMOs will encourage further empire building in medicine, while protecting the already entrenched interests of the major providers of health care. In the following discussion, we consider the latent goals and benefits of NHI and HMOs, before evaluating their potential for obtaining their manifest goals.

LATENT GOALS

Medical schools and teaching hospitals In recent years, expanding medical centers—comprised of medical schools and teaching hospitals—have taken the place of the conservative American Medical Association in dominating the power structure of American medicine. Planners associated with these large medical centers frequently have acted as outspoken advocates for increased government programs and spending for health care. Nevertheless, the medical centers are in trouble. Until the middle 1960's, the federal government and private philanthropies were providing lucrative support for basic science research. Research grants formed a major source of revenues which helped medical empires expand. Then, largely because of the financial pressures imposed by the Indochina War and inflation, research money began to dry up. Sentiment arose that available funds should be used in practical applications of medical knowledge, rather than in further basic research.

The response of major health institutions was swift and dramatic. Many medical schools established departments of community medicine. Others inaugurated new health programs in nearby ghettoes whose severe health problems had gone unnoticed for years. Still others started outreach projects in rural areas. Often these new programs overlapped with each other and competed for patients and funds. Regional planning and control remained negligible.

During the last three years, as the concept of HMOs has become more popular among government granting agencies, medical centers have jumped on the HMO bandwagon. First at Harvard, then at Yale, Johns Hopkins, and Washington University in St. Louis, and more recently at numerous other schools, HMOs have come into existence, attracting significant outside funding. J. V. Maloney, recent president of the American Society of University Surgeons, has commented caustically on the medical schools' newly found enthusiasm for HMOs:

> It is curious that the university whose principal mission is teaching clinical medicine in a scholarly environment should suddenly become interested in the delivery of health care. The answer seems to be that given by Willy Sutton, the often apprehended bank robber, when asked why he insisted on robbing banks: " 'Cause that's where the money is!" The enthusiasm for prepaid health schemes at several universities surveyed was related to the severity of their fiscal crisis and shortage of clinical material (1970:16).

There is little doubt that HMOs are potential money makers. The experience of the first university-affiliated HMO, the Harvard Community Health Plan (HCHP), is typical. Figure 13 shows the changes in govern-

Figure 13. Government and philanthropic receipts of Harvard Medical School (_____) versus Harvard Community Health Plan (_ _ _ _), by year

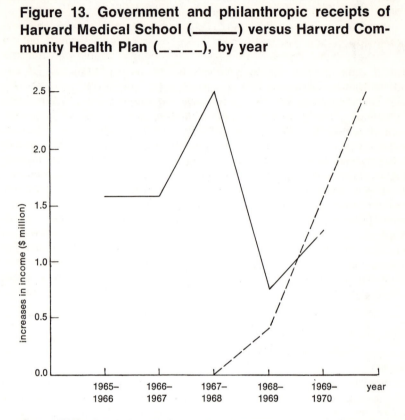

Source: "HMOs: A critical appraisal of the Harvard Community Health Plan" by Howard Waitzkin and Alana S. Cohen, in Harvard Medical Alumni Bulletin 47 (Sept.-Oct. 1972:14). Reprinted courtesy of the publisher, as taken from the financial report to the board of overseers of Harvard College, and Harvard Community Health Plan.

ment and philanthropic grants which Harvard Medical School used from 1965 to 1970. Following a steady increase until 1968, grants began to fall off. Some Harvard teaching hospitals had actual reductions in research funding; in other cases, inflated costs meant that smaller increases in federal support were experienced as net decreases. Harvard's success in attracting funds for its new HMO also is shown in Figure 13. At the same time as federal funding for research has decelerated, government and philanthropic funding of HCHP has increased.

The development of new modes of financing does not imply that Harvard or other medical centers could correct all their financial problems through HMOs. Most money received is restricted for HMO activities; a school could not, for example, transfer funds designated for an HMO to cover expenses for basic research. In addition, for HCHP and similar plans, unexpectedly high costs have created financial difficulties during their first years of operation. At a time of declining revenue for research, however, entry into the HMO field helps Harvard and similar medical empires to preserve their over-all financial strength.

Furthermore, university-affiliated HMOs are now trying to extend services to low-income patients. Again, there is more than altruism behind such moves; providing HMO services to low-income people can become a money-making venture too. All HMOs which have offered care to patients with limited finances have received large federal and philanthropic grants to cover these services; in no case has the provision of care been a matter of "charity medicine." For example, large Office of Economic Opportunity (OEO) awards have gone to Kaiser's programs in Portland, Oregon, and Los Angeles. Another example is that of HCHP, whose largest outside grants have been earmarked for services to low-income patients. In fact, the prepaid capitation fees which HCHP receives for low-income subscribers have been *higher* than those it obtains for wealthier enrollees.

HMO planners doubtless are motivated by a genuine concern about improving health care for the poor. On the other hand, they make sure that their institutions do not incur significant risks in such ventures. For instance, HCHP presently has received almost one million dollars annually for a total projected low-income enrollment of 6,000. As shown in Table 2, HCHP's initial monthly capitation for adults was five to six dollars

Table 2. Monthly capitation per person, Harvard Community Health Plan ($)

Coverage

Private carrier		Medicaid		Supplementation grant	
		Initial	April, 1971	Initial	April, 1971
Adult	17.01	23.87	19.89	23.00	21.00
Child	9.08	12.98	10.82	12.00	11.00
Elderly person	—	22.98	19.15	22.00	20.00

Source: "HMOs: A Critical Appraisal of the Harvard Community Health Plan" by Howard Waitzkin and Alana S. Cohen, in Harvard Medical Alumni Bulletin 47 (Sept.-Oct. 1972):15. Reprinted courtesy of the publisher.

higher for low-income patients (covered by welfare or Public Health Service "supplementation" grants) than for upper-income subscribers (covered by commercial insurance companies or Blue Cross); the comparable figure for children was three to four dollars.

Administrators explain these higher capitations on the basis of a possibly greater risk of illness or injury in the low-income groups. The rationale is that the increment will provide a contingency against the risk of greater utilization of services by these patients.

Despite this theory, a variety of studies have shown that low-income patients actually utilize available health services *less* frequently than other patients. Although the gap in utilization between low-income patients and those with higher incomes has narrowed in recent years (as Medicare and Medicaid assistance has become available) utilization rates of most health services remain lower for the poor (Roghmann et al., 1971; Andersen et al., 1972:33–34 et passim; Aday and Eichhorn, 1972: 22–24; Roemer et al., 1972:20,31; Greenlick et al., 1972). Based on the first year of operation, HCHP officials decided in 1971 that the rate of utilization by low-income subscribers justified a reduction in capitations. The lesser figures, however, still remained higher than for patients covered by commercial insurance carriers (Table 2).

Even the revised capitations meant that HCHP would receive significantly more money for low-income families who were enrolled. For example, as shown in Table 3, annual capitations paid to HCHP for a

---

Table 3. Total annual capitation for family of 7 (2 adults and 5 children). Harvard Community Health Plan ($)*

Coverage

Private carrier	Medicaid	Supplementation grant
953.04	1126.56	1164.00

Source: "HMOs: A Critical Appraisal of the Harvard Community Health Plan" by Howard Waitzkin and Alana S. Cohen, in Harvard Medical Alumni Bulletin 47(Sept.-Oct. 1972):15. Reprinted courtesy of the publisher.

*Rates effective April 1, 1971.

---

low-income family of two adults and five children would total about two hundred dollars more than for upper-income patients.

This type of capitation schedule is typical of the ways by which HMOs can use low-income patients to improve their own monetary position, and indirectly that of their sponsoring institutions. Unless low-income subscribers show markedly higher utilization patterns in the future—an outcome which appears unlikely in view of the experience thus far—HMOs stand to benefit financially by the enrollment of these patients.

The sudden interest in initiating HMO programs for local communities diverts public attention from the central concerns of medical empires; expansion into these spheres provides a new source of revenue while enhancing institutional prestige. Furthermore, HMO programs suggest that their sponsoring medical centers are on the forefront of health care innovations, while allowing the organizations to meet their own internal maintenance and enhancement needs.

Thus, the interest in HMOs extends beyond monetary concerns. HMOs affiliated with medical schools also will help maintain the population of patients available for teaching purposes. Medicare, Medicaid, and other government programs provide hospital accommodations and services for low-income patients which are equivalent to those enjoyed by private patients. People who previously had no alternative to ward medicine, and who, therefore, served as "teaching material" for medical students and house officers, increasingly are able to avoid participation in teaching. The possibility that medical schools will be turning to private patients for teaching has evoked widespread concern among medical educators (Richards, 1971).

Several new HMOs explicitly intend to use HMO patients for teaching. In general, the teaching hospitals associated with HMOs have begun to show declining patient censuses, and the proportion of empty beds at a given time has increased. Therefore, the number of patients who might contribute to teaching has diminished. At these hospitals it is hoped that patients who have been lost from the charity clinics and wards will be replaced by people enrolled in HMOs (e.g., Stanford University School of Medicine, 1972). Officials of some HMOs are aware that in the past many patients have had unpleasant experiences in teaching exercises. As a result, planners have hesitated to introduce teaching functions in the HMOs' initial period of patient care. In these cases, administrators generally plan to expand teaching gradually, after the HMOs become fully accepted by their clientele (Dorsey, 1973).

What difference does it make if HMOs serve the interests of medical empires? The issue would be less critical if the self-interest of such empires did not directly undermine the manifest purposes of HMOs. The establishment of HMOs in close proximity to existing medical centers does little, if anything, to improve the distribution of health care in the country as a whole. It is true that several HMOs have extended services to urban low-income patients, who enjoy easier access to care now than in the past. Still, the disparities are huge and are likely to remain so if medical centers are free to start HMOs on a strictly voluntary basis.

Poor coordination, ineffective regional planning, and continuing maldistribution of health services are the probable outcomes of this process. As an example, two HMOs (HCHP and Health, Inc.—the latter, a group practice which retains fee-for-service rather than prepaid financing) have arisen in affiliation with different Harvard teaching hospitals (cf. Cronkhite et al., 1971; Hiatt, 1971). These two HMOs have competed with each other for local subscribers. Representatives of HCHP and Health, Inc., have approached the same tenants' associations and other groups in Boston with offers of services to members of these organizations. Community residents often speak of "turf battles" between HCHP and Health, Inc. Although low-income people living near the Harvard teaching hospitals have had less trouble in obtaining medical care, patients in other areas of Boston— let alone the medically destitute areas of western Massachusetts and northern New England—continue to have the same old problems.

These trends, which are emerging in cities throughout the country where large medical centers already exist, convey an impression of overlapping and duplicated programs. They are reminiscent of the multiplicity of expensive, technologically advanced facilities (such as radiation therapy and transplantation units) which are also contained within a small geographic area. Although a basic tenet of comprehensive planning is that overlapping facilities should be avoided, this principle does not appear to apply to medical centers' involvement in HMOs. Rather than merging and co-ordinating programs, each institution seems intent on establishing its own plan, even in competition with similar plans sponsored by neighboring hospitals. Maintenance of the financial and power position of each institution—again, the issue of medical imperialism—seems to receive highest priority.

Obviously the country should address the problems of its medical schools, which must have sufficient operating funds and enough informed patients *from all income levels* who willingly agree to participate in teaching. But these problems, together with the problem of maldistribution, will not be solved by the haphazard establishment of HMOs linked to existing medical centers, where personnel and facilities already are heavily concentrated.

Blue Cross and the commercial insurance carriers The insurance industry also has moved rapidly into the HMO field. Metropolitan Life Insurance Company is giving financial support to Washington University's HMO in St. Louis. Connecticut General Life Insurance Company is making a large investment in the HMO affiliated with Johns Hopkins. Ten commercial insurance carriers, in addition to Massachusetts Blue Cross, have agreed to offer HCHP benefits to their subscribers. One of Health, Inc.'s corporate sponsors in Boston is the New England Life Insurance Company.

These insurance companies are bastions of American capitalism. For example, eight of the companies affiliated with HCHP rank among the 26 richest corporations in the United States; their cumulative assets total over 98 billion dollars (Fortune Magazine, 1972). What does the insurance industry stand to gain from its involvement with HMOs?

The insurance companies' profits from existing HMOs actually are quite small. In some cases, insurance companies have given direct financial support to HMOs in the form of grants. In other cases, they have underwritten part of the risk of hospitalization or ambulatory care for HMO patients. For several HMOs, the insurance companies also perform administrative functions, such as billing, receiving payments, processing subscribers' claims, and collecting statistics. Generally, the financial gain to the insurance companies has been limited. At HCHP, for example, the companies receive 4 to 8 percent of the premium dollar. This return represents a small profit, especially when compared to the more lucrative forms of coverage which the commercial carriers sell, both inside and outside the health field.

Viewed from a slightly different perspective, however, participation in HMOs may emerge as an excellent investment for the insurance industry in the long run. Blue Cross and especially the commercial carriers would serve no necessary functional purpose if NHI were enacted. That is, under NHI an independent federal bureaucracy could administer the collection of premiums and payment of benefits without involvement of the present insurance industry.

Yet most proposals for NHI presently under consideration—such as those of the American Medical Association, the Nixon Administration, and the Health Insurance Association of America—would rely on the commercial carriers as an integral part of NHI. Under these plans, insurance companies would assume one of two roles. One possibility is that NHI would merely provide public subsidies for low-income individuals, so that they could buy health insurance through the existing structure. Alternatively, NHI would insure all members of the population, but the present insurance companies would provide the administrative apparatus.

It should be noted, however, that NHI could be established without any participation by the insurance industry. Senator Kennedy's plan, for example, excludes the industry completely. Instead, it substitutes a federal "Health Security Board" with administrative responsibility for NHI (while relying for its revenues on a regressive tax system which resembles Social Security in taxing employees) (Kennedy, 1971: Section G).

Because it need not be part of NHI, the insurance industry must move rapidly to justify its role in any future NHI programs. Neither Blue Cross nor the commercial carriers have achieved exemplary records of innovation. Blue Cross has received criticism throughout the country for rate hikes which contribute to the over-all costs of medical services. Only recently have the commercial carriers begun to argue in favor of comprehensive care in the context of HMOs. It appears that the insurance industry's new interest reflects a need to legitimate its continued existence as a part of the health-care system (cf. Kelman, 1971:34–35).

Since the demand for medical services is virtually limitless, the exclusion of commercial companies from health insurance would imply a considerable financial loss to the insurance industry. Consequently, the industry must be able to present evidence to legislators and the general public that it can play an effective role in the medical care of the future. Since NHI probably will recognize and support HMOs if it is enacted, insurance companies are eager to associate themselves with the HMOs now being formed. Such experience will provide a strong argument that the insurance industry can function as the administrative apparatus of NHI, or as a conduit of NHI money from the government to providers of services.

On the other hand, officials of university-affiliated HMOs acknowledge that an expanded bureaucracy within the HMOs themselves could perform administrative tasks just as efficiently as Blue Cross and the commercial carriers. This fact hardly justifies the profits which may accrue to the insurance industry under NHI.

Why have the new HMOs entered into alliances with the insurance industry? HMOs are yet another means by which the various medical provider institutions can work cooperatively to enhance their respective interests in the name of providing better care. Furthermore, there are several purely pragmatic reasons for these alliances (Pollack, 1968).

First, in many states, HMOs cannot obtain charters to sell insurance under existing state laws. Co-operation with Blue Cross and the insurance companies allows HMOs to circumvent this legal problem.

A second pragmatic reason for involving the insurance companies derives from uncertainty about the future of health-care financing. HMO planners believe that changes in financing will occur, probably in the direction of NHI, but do not know whether the insurance industry will continue to play an active role in new government programs. As a hedge against uncertainty, planners decide to co-operate with the insurance industry because it may form a component of future programs in health-care delivery.

Thirdly, most HMOs must attract subscribers who already hold other forms of insurance. New university-affiliated HMOs often have no readily apparent consumer population comparable to those of other large group practices—such as the employees of Kaiser industries or the labor unions which have sponsored HMOs. Planners anticipate public opposition from the insurance industry if they attempt to operate as independent insurance agencies, taking subscribers away from existing companies. Therefore, to avoid greater difficulty in enrolling patients, new HMOs have entered into agreements by which insurance companies can offer HMO benefits to their own subscribers. Individuals have the option of joining the HMOs, and their premiums are channeled through the same insurance companies. By avoiding acrimony between HMOs and the insurance industry, administrators hope to expand enrollment.

The participation of Blue Cross and the commercial insurance carriers in HMOs, therefore, offers advantages to the insurance industry and to the HMOs. The HMOs pragmatically have based their decisions to cooperate with the industry on several legal, financial, and political gains which planners anticipate. In these decisions, there has been essentially no critical evaluation of the long-term policy implications of this alliance. Yet, especially if the insurance industry serves no demonstrable function under NHI, the question remains whether the industry's future profits from health care are in the public interest, or are merely another example of the exploitation of illness on the part of the medical-industrial complex.

Professional associations Of the medical professional associations, the American Medical Association has been most powerful. In the past it not only has pressured individual physicians into conforming to its ideologies, but also has had an important impact on national health policy. Furthermore, the AMA sets standards for the paraprofessions by controlling their licensing procedures and the accreditation of schools in these areas.

The AMA is famous for its powerful and conservative lobbying efforts. Since the 1930s the AMA has fought against any legislative program that might hint at socialized medicine. In particular, a great deal of expense and energy went into attempts to prevent the passage of Medicare (Harris, 1966). Not only has the AMA been opposed to governmental interference in medicine, but it has fought adamantly for the individual physician's right to private entrepreneurship.

Much surprise has been expressed that the AMA is now in favor of

NHI and HMOs, after its adamant battles against government involvement in health care. However, if examined more closely, this ideological turn-about is understandable in the light of professional self-interest. Because public pressure for change in the health care system is so great, and because of the waning power of this dominant professional association, the AMA has realized that reforms in American medicine are inevitable. Rather than facing the possibility of a thorough re-organization of health care delivery, the AMA—including many of its members—has added its own proposal for NHI-HMOs. As long as health care does not become entirely public, health professionals need not fear government-employed physicians, open medical school enrollment, and governmental licensing and accreditation procedures. In short, the AMA and related professional associations (such as the American College of Physicians, the American Nursing Association, and so on) have come to favor NHI-HMOs because they fear more radical alternatives which might curb professional auton-omy. Similarly, the American Hospital Association would prefer NHI and HMOs to the possibility of strict governmental regulation of hospitals.

As long as NHI-HMOs remain voluntaristic and do not threaten the private nature of American health care delivery, the professional associa-tions are eager to see their realization. Some legislative response to the health crisis is imminent, and these innovations are more palatable to these associations than compulsory measures which would threaten pro-fessional dominance. The idea that doctors should be free to practice as they see fit is deeply ingrained, perhaps because it is linked to basic values like individualism and private enterprise. NHI-HMO proposals have become popular among professional associations chiefly because they will not threaten professional autonomy.

Businesses offering HMO benefits to employees Finally it is interesting to note the advantages NHI-HMOs will offer other large businesses not directly involved in the health industry. Throughout the country, many companies are stating their willingness to pay their employees' premiums for HMO enrollment. These organizations' interest in HMOs is more com-plex than simple concern for their employees' health, and this issue deserves brief comment.

A company's provision of health care is a fringe benefit, that is, a form of non-income compensation. Employees otherwise would spend a por-tion of their annual income for medical care on a fee-for-service basis. Therefore, the purchase of health care by employers results in an effec-tive increase in employees' compensation.

Employers need not pay Social Security or related taxes on this non-income compensation. Similarly, health care received as a fringe benefit is excluded from individual income taxes, according to Internal Revenue Service regulations (U.S. Internal Revenue Service, 1970: Section 1.106–1). As a result of these advantages, HMOs enable employers to increase employees' effective compensation without the expense of higher taxes.

On the surface, the provision of health care as a fringe benefit appears to hurt nobody. As S. M. Miller and Pamela Roby have shown, however, non-monetary compensation increases the inequalities between the many poor, unorganized workers who do not receive fringe benefits and the rest of the labor force (1970:52–56). From trends so far, it appears that upper-income workers are most likely to receive HMO benefits from employers. Perhaps more important, the financial implications of offering health services as a fringe benefit have led to a further commercialization of medical care. Rather than viewing health services as a basic right of the sick, corporate executives favor participation in HMOs because of their financial advantages.

NHI-HMOs serve the interests of different sectors of the American health system in different ways. However, the latent goals of these innovations can be summarized quite simply: *NHI and HMOs will preserve the present distribution of power within American medicine.* Since this distribution of power already has created a crisis in health care (Lasker, 1971), it is dubious that real change will occur while the providers of health care retain control. Until the balance of power is shifted from health providers toward consumers, the ongoing priorities of medical imperialism will predominate over the needs of patients. NHI-HMOs will continue to foster the empire building which has become characteristic of American medicine. Imperialism in health care will not be stayed unless the medical-industrial hegemony gives way to a more egalitarian exchange of influence and control between consumers and providers of health care. NHI and HMOs do not in any way point in this direction; instead, they portend maintenance of the status quo. The enactment of NHI-HMO legislation may avert more basic changes in the organization of health care which could topple the medical-industrial complex.

MANIFEST GOALS

More important, NHI and HMOs may also fall short of the manifest goals for which they are to be established. These goals, as cited above, include improved distribution, reduced costs, and enhanced quality of medical services. In evaluating the potential contribution of HMOs under NHI, we shall review HMOs' accomplishments from the standpoint of these goals.

Distribution NHI does not imply re-organization of the present health system. Financial incentives under NHI might encourage physicians to serve in areas which lack sufficient medical personnel and facilities. NHI by no means guarantees, however, that patients in medically deprived areas will enjoy greater access to care. Potentially NHI may equalize patients' ability to pay, while not affecting the inaccessibility of medical services for much of the population.

Even proponents of NHI realize that it will not rectify the inequalities inherent in contemporary American health care. For example, the economist Rashi Fein has argued in behalf of NHI because it will create such a crisis that the public will demand needed changes in the organization of services:

> *I think that it's healthier to have the queues, to have people frustrated [under NHI], so that we see that there are people who are not getting medical care because of a shortage of physicians, or because of lack of organization. I don't want to cover it up. . . . If we institute a national health insurance system, there will be strains, there will be pressures. But I do not think that the American system will legislate changes first, and I am willing to push for national insurance because I think that this will force us to address the problem of change (Fein, 1970:171).*

From this viewpoint, NHI would lead to another crisis in health care, rather than resolving the present crisis.

If NHI is enacted, the probability is high that *millions of dollars will be wasted because of the mistaken impression that changes in financing imply changes in organizational structure.* Instead, this money will even more firmly entrench the expanding medical empires and their business partners. While medical centers increase their prestige and power, and the medical industry its profits, many Americans will remain without adequate health care.

HMOs, like NHI, do not guarantee any systematic re-organization of the health system. Again, they are latently functional for the providers of medical services. To date, HMOs have not proved themselves to be advantageous to medical patients in terms of achieving the goals for which they are manifestly conceived.

Low-income people rarely have benefitted from HMOs. The vast majority of prepaid group practices now in existence are located in upper-income areas of cities and in suburbs where there is little shortage of health personnel. Only a few HMOs have served patients with limited finances, and these have been primarily cases in which federal agencies have awarded grants to HMOs intending to enroll low-income people (Greenberg and Rodburg, 1971; Columbo et al., 1969; Greenlick et al., 1972).

In addition to these few attempts to increase the availability of health care for the poor, some HMOs have tried to improve geographical distribution. A handful of HMOs have arisen in small cities (for example, the Marshfield Clinic in Wisconsin) and rural areas (the HMO in Two Harbors, Minnesota).

The voluntaristic assumptions on which HMOs are based, however, do not assure that all low-income people or patients living in rural areas will receive HMO services. As already described, the formation of HMOs serving low-income patients is creating a new form of grantsmanship, which will benefit medical schools and large hospitals. Low-income people who happen to live close to these institutions may receive better medical care, but there is no guarantee that HMOs will increase services to the low-income urban population at large.

Even more haphazard will be the effects of HMOs in rural areas. In some parts of Appalachia, the South, and the Midwest, the ratio of physicians to patients is about 40 per 100,000 as compared to a national average of about 150 per 100,000 (Appalachian Region Health Policy and Planning Council, 1969:103). Because of rural poverty, population dispersal, and the unavailability of referral centers, practice in these areas is extremely difficult. Cultural and education advantages for physicians and their families also are lacking.

Although NHI may provide financial incentives for rural HMOs, it is difficult to see how these incentives will be sufficient to attract large numbers of health workers. Again the question arises whether voluntary mechanisms, like the establishment of HMOs, will solve rural health problems.

Costs Proponents of HMOs have claimed that the prepaid approach can reduce the costs of health care. Theoretically, HMOs could lower costs through two mechanisms. First, since prepaid coverage provides comprehensive outpatient services, it tends to decrease the number and length of subscribers' hospitalizations. These effects on hospitalizations have been observed consistently in the HMOs established so far and are often cited as convincing evidence of cost reduction.

A second argument holds that HMOs which control their own hospitals, such as Kaiser, experience internal pressures toward efficiency. Since HMOs' income from premiums is the same regardless of the number or duration of hospitalizations, there is an incentive to decrease hospitalization time and to improve efficiency within hospitals. This situation differs from Blue Cross-Blue Shield or commercial health insurance plans, which reimburse hospitals at a standardized schedule for services and which often encourage hospitalization by excluding coverage for outpatient care. Individual doctors who belong to HMOs also try to reduce hospitalizations, since their salaries increase to the extent that expenses for hospitalization and maintenance costs can be minimized.

Although most existing HMOs report less hospitalization, there is little evidence that HMOs will significantly cut the over-all costs of medical care. Also, it is doubtful that cost cutting by reduced hospitalization is wholly desirable. The Kaiser Plan in California has produced data showing costs 20 to 30 percent lower than outside the Plan. Kaiser has received criticism, however, concerning its attempts to control costs by restricting hospitalization. Patients requiring elective admissions to Kaiser hospitals have experienced long delays. To avoid such inconveniences, many subscribers have used facilities or personnel outside the Plan (Moore and Bodenheimer, 1973; Carnoy, 1970; cf. Somers, 1971). In other HMOs, especially those which try to enroll low-income people, numerous patients turn to doctors and hospitals outside the HMOs to receive part of their care. The cost of services obtained outside an HMO, of course, does not enter into the computation of the HMO's total costs.

Another factor which casts doubt on HMOs' cost-cutting potential is the large initial capital investment which is necessary. Capital needs for the establishment of an HMO are huge. In university-affiliated HMOs, initial outlay amounts to several million dollars. This expenditure is followed by a period of two to three years of deficit accounting (usually covered by outside grants) until subscribers' premiums balance the HMO's maintenance costs.

Furthermore, the conditions and clientele of HMOs vary considerably. In plans like Kaiser, which serve predominantly upper-income executives and workers, patients for the most part were receiving adequate care prior to joining the HMO. On the other hand, low-income patients, who have not obtained sufficient services previously, may have a backlog of unattended health problems. This backlog would tend to increase the services an HMO would have to provide if it enrolled low-income people and if those people utilized the services which were available. The variability in the conditions under which HMOs are established may account for several studies which have found either a minimal or negligible cost reduction by new HMOs (Greenberg and Rodburg, 1971).

In summary, despite HMOs' ability to reduce the frequency and duration of hospitalizations, the evidence that HMOs alone will decrease and control the over-all costs of medical care is inconsistent and unconvincing.

Quality The issue of quality always holds a central place in arguments for HMOs. HMOs allow for teamwork—a group of doctors, nurses, and allied health personnel who can consult with each other when different specialty services are needed. The medical care an HMO provides is comprehensive and often preventive. Patients can make appointments at will to be seen as outpatients. By preventive screening, the HMO can theoretically preserve health rather than merely reacting to illness episodes. Because a single prepaid fee covers all services, HMOs can provide continuity of care.

Proponents of HMOs also believe that the group relationship itself enhances the quality of services provided. Since health professionals work in close proximity, peer review would assure the competence of each individual practitioner. The group context also would encourage continuing medical education. Doctors and other personnel could hold conferences, discuss recent literature, substitute for one another if a practitioner chose to attend a postgraduate medical course, and so forth.

All these theoretical advantages of HMOs sound attractive. On closer inspection, however, one finds that they are more theoretical than real. Quality of health care is an extremely difficult parameter to measure. Although HMOs have decreased hospitalization, this fact in itself does not necessarily reflect improved quality. In HMOs, problems which otherwise would be approached by hospitalizing a patient often are handled on an outpatient basis. But this does not mean that illness or deaths among HMO patients are declining.

No HMO has yet been able to show an improvement in the mortality (death rate) or morbidity (rate of illness episodes) among its patients as opposed to a comparable control group of patients not enrolled in

HMOs. In fact, several disappointing studies of comprehensive care programs (when compared to episodic care in fee-for-service private practice, in hospital clinics, or in emergency rooms) recently have demonstrated no improvements in morbidity, mortality, or other indices reflecting the outcomes of care (Gordis and Markowitz, 1971; Moore et al., 1972).

Have HMOs improved the more subjective, and less readily measurable, aspects of medicine—such as patient satisfaction? Several existing HMOs have encountered severe criticism from consumers about poor quality. Patients of the Health Insurance Plan of New York, for example, have complained about lack of privacy during physical examinations, inability to get the doctor they wanted, long waits to see a doctor, and difficulties in obtaining emergency services (Schwartz, 1972; Levy and Fein, 1972: 16; cf. Moore and Bodenheimer, 1973).

Most theoretical benefits of HMOs actually reflect the ideological preferences of current health planners who represent the present power structure of American medicine. It seems reasonable that modifications in the organization of practice, encouraging the formation of groups, will improve quality. But this idea has never been proven by observed changes in morbidity, mortality, or other health measures. In addition, HMOs often do not realize their potential for consultation, peer review, and continuing medical education. Observations of actual HMOs have shown that quality review tends to be negligible or irregular. If HMOs cannot be shown to improve the health of their own subscribers, and if the establishment of HMOs is to remain purely voluntary, one cannot assume that HMOs will beneficially affect the health of the population at large.

In summary, therefore, the evidence does not justify the claims made by proponents of NHI and HMOs. Both innovations fall short of ensuring reorganization of the health system. Instead, the viability of these plans depends on the good will of health workers and the network of organizations that provide medical services in this country. However, as has been discussed, NHI and HMOs are essentially conservative rather than progressive innovations. While there is no promise that these plans will significantly change health care delivery, it is clear that they will tend to enhance medical imperialism. Offered as a panacea to the health crisis, these innovations will more likely perpetuate exploitation of patients by maintaining the ongoing power distribution in American medicine.

Finally, one may contrast NHI and HMOs with the outcomes that would accompany a national health service (NHS). The most crucial distinction between NHI-HMO proposals and NHS concerns the issue of voluntarism. Under NHI, doctors remain free to determine the location and type of practice they prefer. NHI only guarantees that they will be paid for services they provide to patients, not that they must practice in areas of shortage. Similarly, plans for HMOs do not include the mandatory establishment of HMOs throughout the country; doctors will retain autonomy in deciding whether to enter group practice.

Under an NHS, since physicians are employees of government, they can be assigned to areas of need, often on a rotating basis. In many countries where health facilities previously were maldistributed, an NHS has greatly increased the availability of medical services. The establishment of an NHS implies a *re-organization* of the health system, rather than simply changes in financing. The NHS, unlike NHI-HMOs, achieves this effect largely through *compulsory* measures.

Beyond reduction of distributional inequalities, an NHS also limits costs by controlling doctors' salaries and enforcing limits on hospital expenditures—two of the most rapidly rising components of health costs since the enactment of Medicare and Medicaid. The problem of assessing quality would remain; one should note, however, that countries served by some form of NHS generally have low rates of infant mortality and high life expectancy (United Nations, 1972a:76–80).

Compulsory mechanisms would not automatically solve all the nation's health problems. Depersonalization, alienation, and bureaucratic inefficiencies continue to exist in national health services, and any system which treats illness reinforces the sick role, which lends support to the status quo.

On the other hand we consider compulsory mechanisms to be a requisite first step in the development of a medical system that guarantees citizens their right to health care. As a first stage, centralization of health planning is crucial in assuring that all regions of the country receive the facilities and personnel that are needed. Centralization would make it possible to allocate larger health expenditures for areas which previously have been deprived of care. Thus a pattern for health services in the entire country would be accomplished.

However, the initial centralization of medical planning eventually would need to be offset by increasing decentralization. That is, individual communities—including patients and health personnel—would implement programs on a local level. After a time, local determination of health needs presumably would supersede centralized planning as the major political process by which medical services would be delivered to each indivdual in the country.

We suggest that a dialectic between centralization, with compulsory redistribution, and decentralization, with cooperative self-determination, could culminate in a new form for delivering health care. A health system organized according to essentially anarchist principles could be successful only if it followed a compulsory redistribution of personnel and facilities. Such a system would be comprised of small communities in which consumers and providers would work together to ensure each individual's right to medical care.

The evolution of such a system would not be accomplished without a great deal of political struggle—a struggle in which patients would have definitive impact on all levels of planning, implementation, and evaluation. This type of public health system will be outlined further in the next chapter. It should be noted, however, that such a system would eliminate medical imperialism and, more specifically, the exploitation of illness on which it is based.

6 Toward a Nonexploitative Health System

Is a humane health care system possible in a capitalist society?

No is a simplistic answer, but certainly a logical conclusion of this study. The institution of medicine is intimately connected to other social institutions. In capitalist societies, illness is exploited for a variety of purposes while medical services remain inadequate. The sick role offers a conservative and in some cases counterrevolutionary mechanism by which people in trouble can deviate temporarily from their usual roles. Meanwhile, the social control functions of the sick role reduce the potentiality for organized opposition against structural injustices in society. Health care is one dimension by which a population is stratified in capitalist societies. Moreover, professionalism, elitism, and restricted communication foster stratification within the institution of medicine itself. Illness forms the basis of medical imperialism by large organizations such as medical schools and university-affiliated hospitals, whose expansion often interferes with the non-medical needs of low-income people. By all indications, health maintenance organizations and national health insurance will exacerbate the problem of empire building, without correcting the fundamental maldistribution of health personnel and facilities.

One cannot contemplate modifications in the health system isolated from the broader social system of which it is a part. The United States presently spends 40 to 50 percent of its gross national product on defense and associated industries, while health and welfare receive less than 20 percent of federal allocations (U.S., Department of Commerce, 1972:384–385; cf. Titmuss, 1971). Massive economic conversion away from capital-intensive enterprise related to defense is a precondition for any serious re-orientation of health and welfare on a societal scale. Though widely advocated, economic conversion is becoming a more elusive reality. In this section, we briefly discuss several programmatic requirements for a humanistic, non-alienating, nonexploitative health system. We do so, however, with a somewhat jaundiced eye, perceiving the utopian nature of our suggestions within the context of contemporary American social structure (cf. Medical Committee for Human Rights, 1972: 117–122).

Profits from illness must be abolished Profiteering reflects exploitation in its most egregious form. In fee-for-service medicine, private practitioners are able to earn exorbitant incomes, far in excess of their needs. Moreover, capitalist industries have shown great ingenuity in extracting profit from the vulnerability of individuals suffering ill health. The chance occurrence of illness in the American population leads to profits for several industries: insurance companies, pharmaceutical firms, medical equipment and supply houses, corporations managing private nursing homes, proprietary hospitals, and so forth. So-called non-profit hospitals support the profit structure of the "medical-industrial complex" by duplicating advanced technological facilities without regional coordination. Non-profit hospitals frequently have overlapping directorships with profit-making health industries, the managers and owners of which often serve on hospitals' boards of directors (Lasker, 1971). In addition to supporting industries whose explicit goal is profit from illness, patients must also sustain the largely unnecessary overhead expenses of non-profit hospitals, especially those expenses related to research not contributing directly to patient care.

Profits from illness have no place in a nonexploitative health system. This principle has several implications for change, if an evaluative decision is made to create a health system responsive to the needs of patients in the United States. First, industries manufacturing products such as drugs and medical equipment should be nationalized. In fact, nationalization of the medical-industrial complex appears to be the only reasonable means by which patients will no longer bear the excess costs of illness. Second, private insurance companies should be permitted no role in health care. Instead, all members of society should pay for health care through a progressive taxation structure. Through this mechanism, economic considerations would cease to be a disincentive for low-income patients' seeking care on a regular basis—rather than only in times of acute illness. Likewise, added profits to the insurance industry would no longer comprise a major portion of patients' health expenses.

Third, private fee-for-service practice should be eliminated. As previously discussed, the "sliding scale" has proved itself to be notoriously erratic in the delivery of adequate health care to low-income patients. All physicians should receive a decent income. However, their employer should be some level of government—local, state, or federal. The details of such employment might depend on the conditions in which doctors practice. (The potentialities of a national health service in the United States are considered later in this section.) Because economic incentives under the fee-for-service principle would be irrelevant to salaried physicians, they presumably would respond more equitably to patients of all income levels. The elimination of profits in medical care would not necessarily remove economic problems from the health system. It would, however, shift the financial burden of illness more progressively throughout the population as a whole.

The problem of bureaucracy must be surmounted Any attempt to construct a coordinated public health system would involve the formation of a bureaucracy organized on a national level. The dehumanizing and alienating manifestations of bureaucracy have made themselves felt in many socialist countries which have tried to establish effective health care systems (Weinerman, 1969; Waterman, 1971). As a result, patients often must face cumbersome procedures which inhibit their ability to obtain the health care they seek. Bureaucratic obstacles to adequate health care arise primarily at two points: over-centralization of policy making and inefficient referral networks.

Centralized planning can produce health systems which are rational on paper but ineffective in reality. Each region of a nation experiences unique health problems, which relate to such variables as the dominant economic enterprises, terrain and transportation, degree of urbanization, and so forth. Rural areas which are organized around agriculture, for example, show an incidence of occupational diseases and difficulties of access to medical facilities which differ markedly from those of urban districts with predominantly industrial enterprise. Several Eastern European countries have constructed health systems which, in practice, fail to take into account such local variations. As a result, particularly in rural areas, patients encounter severe inconveniences in obtaining needed services, despite national policies which make health care theoretically available to all citizens (Waterman, 1971). Clearly, a centralized bureaucracy will have difficulties in planning adequately for the diverse needs of an entire population.

A second bureaucratic problem arising in nationally organized health systems concerns the availability of general practitioners, as opposed to specialists. To cite the Yugoslavian example, local health centers are staffed predominantly by general practitioners, who must see a large number of patients each day (Waterman, 1971; cf. Weinerman, 1969). Specialists are available in provincial areas but spend most of their time at large provincial hospitals. Patients with non-emergent conditions who require specialty attention must wait long periods of time and travel long distances to obtain care at these hospitals. Because the separation of general versus specialty services is fairly rigid, difficulties arise at both the local and provincial levels. For patients whose conditions fall within the competence of general practitioners at local health centers, medical care tends to be brief and perfunctory. For problems requiring specialists, patients face inconvenient delay and geographic inaccessibility; their care at the provincial hospitals tends to be impersonal. In short, in countries where health services are organized mainly along bureaucratic lines, the balance of general and specialty services tends to be poorly matched to the specific health needs of local patient populations.

The problem of bureaucracy emerges in any attempt to formulate a framework for a nonexploitative health system. Its solution does not lie in the simple assertion that bureaucratic forms be minimized. Some mechanism must evolve through which planning—particularly involving the allocation of resources and personnel—can occur on a national level. Such a mechanism would inevitably involve some degree of bureaucratic organization. It is a fallacy to believe, as some have argued, that bureaucracy itself necessarily leads to an alienating, cumbersome health system (Halberstam, 1971). As illustrated by health systems in Eastern Europe, bureaucracy exerts its worst effects when it interferes with the day-to-day activities of specific localities, rather than limiting itself to the setting of national goals. From this view, the problem of bureaucracy becomes an issue of central versus local control.

National goals, local control The role of a centralized bureaucracy in a nonexploitative health system need not be complex. In fact, its functions would be predominantly economic. First, a nation must determine on a federal level the priority which health care is to receive within a spectrum of national goals. This decision, basically evaluative, leads directly to budgetary implications. For example, the relatively small proportion of the national budget devoted to health activities in the United States reflects the evaluative priorities of central decision makers. Continued support of the military and related industries reflects policy preferences of the nation's leadership. Redirection of priorities at a national level is a necessary precondition for a humane health system. In brief, *national goals* must be redirected, to recognize the importance of the population's health and welfare needs. With a redirection of national goals, fundamental changes would ensue in the central budgetary processes. Presumably, resources which now are allocated to capital-intensive, defense-related industries would become available in the health sector.

Following these awesome modifications in national priorities, a central bureaucracy's formal functions might be fairly simple, at least in theory. The major goal of such a national organization would be to insure each citizen's right to health care. With a suitable budget, therefore, the bureaucracy's principal tasks would pertain to the distribution of resources. Money made available by a structure of progressive taxation would be distributed to local health institutions according to a formula based on local health needs. A variety of specific formulae might be imagined. One reasonable suggestion is that funds distributed to specific health centers or hospitals be determined by the number of patients using those institutions, and that communities with greater prior needs (i.e., higher rates of illness, lower average income, and so forth) receive somewhat greater initial funding (Medical Committee for Human Rights, 1972:120–121). The crucial point is that the scope of central bureaucratic activities would be quite limited. Once national priorities were re-aligned, a centralized bureaucracy would not play a major role in health policy. Nor would it control the day-to-day activities of local health facilities. The bureaucracy's major task, which theoretically could be accomplished with a relatively small number of personnel, would be the distribution of funds from a central collecting point to the health centers and hospitals which actually provide care.

Local control over health policy would circumvent the problems of a more extensive federal bureaucracy whose uniform procedures tend not to accommodate the variable needs of different groups and localities. Although local control is a problematic topic, its broad directions may be outlined based on the examples of countries in which it has proven effective—particularly Cuba and the People's Republic of China.

Because they are best acquainted with local health needs and working conditions, consumers and health workers would unite to form coalitions responsible for the policies of specific hospitals or health centers. Optimally, as in the case of Cuba and China, councils of workers and consumers would be elected through democratic procedures. On the local level, these councils would control health centers or hospitals—hiring personnel, constructing budgets, determining the type and scope of services provided, and so forth. To coordinate services on a regional level, each local council would elect representatives to a regional council. The regional council would make decisions about hospital expansion and new construction, the establishment and location of technically advanced and specialized facilities (radiation therapy, transplantation teams, etc.), and other matters which affect the availability of services throughout the region. The restriction of medical imperialism would comprise one important goal of the regional council. From this view, tendencies of individual hospitals to expand by establishing duplications of nearby specialty facilities would be sharply curtailed.

The specific details of consumer-worker control need not be rigidly defined. In fact, effective local governance would depend in part on flexibility in establishing decision-making structures appropriate to the needs of different localities (Medical Committee for Human Rights, 1972:120–121). For example, local health councils could contain variable proportions of consumers' and workers' representatives. In communities with significant ethnic or racial minorities, special arrangements might be made to encourage representation from these minorities. Moreover, special groupings could provide the basis for particularistic health facilities, such as women's clinics or health centers for migrant workers. In these cases, the composition of local health councils could be modified to take into account the unique needs of the clinics' clientele.

There are several obvious problems inherent in this projected scheme of consumer-worker control. Perhaps the most significant is the expansionary tendency of all bureaucracies. Although the initial intention might be a limited bureaucracy whose principal function pertains to the distribution of economic resources, encroachment by bureaucrats into the policy affairs of local health councils would be an omnipresent problem requiring constant scrutiny (Downs, 1967). Also, the widely recognized tendency toward oligarchy might limit the true effectiveness of local control. In most democratic organizations, a leadership emerges which often grows distant from the constituency it represents (Michels, 1962). Furthermore, especially in relationships with the professional providers of medical services, local health councils could become objects of co-optation, providing legitimation for decisions which actually would continue to be made by a professional elite (cf. Selznick, 1966). Finally, local control would not necessarily guarantee that the conservative effects of the sick role would be reduced.

These potential problems, however, do not undermine the basic premise of consumer-worker control as a desirable goal. In countries which have assigned high priority to the health and welfare needs of the population, local control has proven an obtainable reality. Beyond issues of policy-making, however, two problems remain. First, how does a country distribute health personnel to areas where they are needed? Second, what kind of authority relations are appropriate within the institution of medicine?

The dialectic between compulsory and voluntary health systems   In Section 5 we discussed health maintenance organizations (HMOs) and national health insurance (NHI)—the two proposed organizational reforms currently in vogue as possible solutions to the crisis in American medicine. As we pointed out, both these proposals remain voluntaristic in nature. Although physicians may be offered financial incentives to practice in areas of severe need, there is no guarantee that areas now lacking adequate facilities and personnel will receive them if HMOs and NHI are enacted. In short, HMOs and NHI will not necessarily correct the distributional problems of American medicine.

By contrast, we considered the potentialities of a national health service (NHS), which uses compulsory mechanisms to distribute health personnel to areas of shortage. Under an NHS, physicians and paraprofessionals are employees of some level of government. As such, they may be assigned— for rotating periods of one to two years—to rural areas and urban districts which experience severe shortages of health workers. For a variety of reasons already discussed, the notion of an NHS has not gained support among any group of American health workers or consumers. However, because of the deeply engrained principle of individualism within the profession of medicine, and because of physicians' dependency on large medical centers which contemporary training programs foster, we doubt that any voluntaristic mechanisms will result in a significant redistribution of personnel.

Compulsory measures are never attractive. One would like to believe that health workers, aware of shortages throughout the country, would go where they are needed. Historically, such a process has not occurred in countries whose health systems have relied on voluntaristic principles. It is a misguided hope that distributional inequalities can be rectified by depending on the good intentions of individual health workers.

On the other hand, we believe that the modifications undertaken in certain socialist countries, especially Cuba and the People's Republic of China, illustrate a dialectic between compulsory and voluntaristic health systems. In both countries, voluntaristic health systems existed prior to the revolutions which established socialism as a unifying governmental principle. These pre-revolutionary systems were highly exploitative. Wealthy patients in urban centers enjoyed high-quality health care, while low-income patients in rural areas and many urban districts could not obtain decent services.

The social revolutions in both Cuba and China brought in their wake the initiation of compulsory mechanisms for redistribution (Horn, 1969; Sidel, 1972; Butler, 1969; John et al., 1971; Medical Committee for Human Rights, 1970; Navarro, 1972). In Cuba young physicians, whose education is totally funded by the government, are expected to serve for at least two years in provincial hospitals or health centers before they are permitted to proceed to specialty training. In China, the government has made extensive efforts to train indigenous paraprofessionals, the "barefoot doctors," to practice in their own communities. Physicians associated with urban medical centers, moreover, are expected to rotate for variable periods of time through the more isolated regions of the country. Their primary function in these rotations is consultative and educational, bringing new knowledge and skills to the paraprofessionals who serve as primary physicians. In addition, the intermittent exposure of all Chinese physicians to the practice of primary medicine keeps them constantly cognizant of the health needs of the Chinese people.

An interesting phenomenon has occurred in both China and Cuba as a concomitant of these compulsory redistributional measures. It has been found that many physicians initially required to practice in provincial areas later choose to remain there, even after they are no longer compelled to do so. These individuals become attached to the communities they serve, find that the problems with which they deal are challenging, and—perhaps because they have not grown dependent on large medical centers—believe that their medical training is appropriate for the tasks at hand. In other words, compulsory health systems in both countries have tended to evolve back to voluntaristic ones, in which physicians continue to serve in areas of need not by compulsion but by free choice.

The anarchist vision of self-sufficient local communities, meeting the needs of the people through systems of mutual aid and voluntary co-operation, does not seem entirely utopian in this context (Kropotkin, 1972a, 1972b; cf. Woodcock, 1962). It is doubtful that the problem of maldistribution in the United States will be solved by the incentives of HMOs and NHI. The problem's scope is too great to rely on voluntaristic principles, which ultimately are based on the highly variable motivations of individual practitioners. On the other hand, an NHS employing compulsory redistributional mechanisms may be an intermediate step between a voluntaristic system which does not meet the needs of the people and one which does.

In this sense, the compulsory nature of an NHS may be viewed as part of a dialectic, by which an exploitative voluntaristic system changes to a nonexploitative voluntaristic system. It seems clear that voluntaristic measures alone will not solve the distributional crisis. Compulsory mechanisms not only may help rectify distributional inequalities but also may represent a transition to a state in which compulsion no longer is necessary. In the United States (which already has required physicians to serve the military through conscription) it is time to consider the advantages of an NHS more seriously.

"Where there is authority there is no freedom": the problem of medical stratification This famous anarchist slogan bears relevance to the problem of stratification within the institution of medicine—a problem more subtle in substance and perhaps more difficult in solution than those discussed above. As pointed out in Section 4, medical stratification is grounded largely in professionalism, elitism, and restricted communication. The detrimental effects of stratification will be resolved only as these issues are addressed forthrightly.

There is some evidence that boundaries of professionalism in the United States are gradually receding. Nurse practitioners are taking on increasing responsibility in patient management, which formerly was the province of physicians (Connally et al., 1966; Lewis and Resnik, 1967). Paraprofessionals are receiving instruction in various programs to function as "physician assistants" (Sox, Sox, and Tompkins, 1973; Carlson and Athelson, 1970; Robert and Tasser, 1970; Kadish and Long, 1970).

Truly basic changes in professionalism will emerge only when professional roles themselves become less reified and training programs more flexible. The traditional four-year medical school and academic medical centers for internship and residency programs are not wholly appropriate educational settings to train health workers whose ultimate function will be primary care. Especially from the example of the People's Republic of China, one concludes that training programs of quite variable length are adequate to provide primary health workers for areas lacking services.

Perhaps more importantly, the hierarchical structures which separate health workers from one another must change. The roles of orderly, physician, nurse, and aide—as well as the ancillary service roles like x-ray and laboratory technician, inhalation therapist, and so forth—should become less differentiated. Patient rounds might be made in common so that all members of the health team participate in therapeutic decision making. Periods of time might be set aside when roles are exchanged: for example, physicians could assume the functions of orderlies or nurses, or the latter could share responsibility with doctors in their work. Through such mechanisms, the rigid walls which divide health workers from each other and which reinforce professionalism would fall.

At present, elitism is a powerful force which inhibits health workers from serving in areas of greatest need. Medical students receive encouragement to pursue internship and residency programs at prestigious medical centers. As training becomes more specialized, these centers become umbilical cords, ultimately preventing doctors from practicing where less technological hardware is available. Criteria for admission to medical school have become extremely complex; in fact, a numerical majority of medical school applicants, though meeting minimum admission requirements, are rejected (American Medical News, 1971; Dube et al., 1971). One infers that the attributes which result in admission pertain less to basic competence in pursuing health studies than to the "gravy" (scientific accomplishments, extra-curricular activities, and so forth) which applicants can present to admission committees.

Two directions of change might ameliorate these tendencies toward elitism. First, an attempt should be made to equalize the resources and personnel available at medical centers throughout the country. This does not necessarily mean downgrading those centers which presently command abundant financial resources and outstanding faculty members, but rather that an attempt should be made to encourage the development of facilities and teaching staffs at medical schools in other geographical areas. Again, such innovations would depend on a central evaluative decision to make financial resources available for health care as opposed to other sectors of the economy. Only through such a decision will young physicians be motivated to obtain postgraduate training at the many American hospitals which presently cannot attract enough interns and residents.

Second, restrictive admission standards to medical schools must be liberalized; this liberalization should be combined with a continued expansion of paraprofessional training. Like the development of training centers for interns and residents, increased medical school admissions also depend on a national evaluative decision about financial resources. New and existing medical schools must receive sufficient funding to permit enlarged enrollments. As a variety of schools augment resources available for teaching, the attractiveness of one school versus another for medical education would diminish. Elitism would wane as the spectrum of strongly staffed, financially viable teaching centers increases.

Finally, stratification within the doctor-patient relationship itself should become less severe. This goal is perhaps the most difficult to attain, since it depends most on the vicissitudes of interpersonal relations. One route to a destratified doctor-patient-relationship, however, would involve a change in restricted communication. The creation of a new paramedical role (discussed in Section 4), the "patient-advocate," could alleviate this problem. Insofar as such an individual would mediate information transmitted from physician to patient by further explanation about illness and possible therapies, the power of doctor over patient would be attenuated. Thus, a more egalitarian doctor-patient relationship would be created, since patients' participation in therapeutic decision making would be based on truly informed consent.

A nonexploitative health system ultimately would be no better than the nonexploitative interactions between individual doctors and individual patients. Improvements in the health system on a larger scale will lack meaning if stratification within doctor-patient relationships themselves is not also reduced. In addition to changes in the broader health system, overcoming exploitation ultimately involves a process of mutual education, by which health workers and patients would come to understand each other's suffering and gladness, pain and satisfaction, fear and sense of accomplishment.

References

Aday, Lu Ann and Robert Eichhorn
1972   "The utilization of health services: indices and correlates." U.S., Department of Health, Education, and Welfare Publications No. (HSM) 73-3003.

Alford, Robert
1972 "The political economy of health care: dynamics without change." Politics and Society 2:127–164.

American Medical Association
1972 Directory of Approved Internships and Residencies, 1972–1973. Chicago: The Association.

American Medical News
1971 "Study of medical school applicants." August 30, page 1.

Andersen, Ronald et al.
1972 "Health service use: national trends and variations." U.S., Department of Health, Education, and Welfare Publications No. (HSM) 73-3004.

Angel, Jerome
1971 The Radical Therapist. New York: Ballantine.

Appalachian Region Health Policy and Planning Council
1969 The Health Development Plan. Greenville, S.C.: The Council.

Arrow, K. J.
1963 "Uncertainty and the welfare economics of medical care." American Economic Review 53:941–973.

Banfield, Edward
1961 Political Influence. New York: Free Press.

Baran, Paul A. and Paul M. Sweezy
1966 Monopoly Capital. New York: Monthly Review Press.

Bell, Daniel
1972 "Lectures on Marxism." Department of Sociology, Harvard University.

Bendix, Reinhard
1969 Nation Building and Citizenship. New York: Anchor.

Bernstein, Basil
1961 "Language and social class." British Journal of Sociology 11:271–276.
1962a "Linguistic codes, hesitation phenomena and intelligence." Language and Speech 5:31–46.
1962b "Social class, linguistic codes and grammatical elements." Language and Speech 5:221–240.
1964a "Elaborated and restricted codes: their social origins and some consequences." American Anthropologist 66 (6):55–69.
1964b "Social class, speech systems and psycho-therapy." British Journal of Sociology 15:54–64.

Bethune, Norman
1969 "Wounds." In "Away With All Pests . . .": An English Surgeon in People's China, by Joshua S. Horn. New York: Monthly Review Press.

Bodenheimer, T. S.
1969 "Regional medical programs: no road to regionalization." Medical Care Review 26:1125–1166.

Bodenheimer, Tom et al.
1972 Billions for Band-aids. San Francisco: Medical Committee for Human Rights.

Boston Women's Health Book Collective
1973 Our Bodies, Our Selves. New York: Simon and Schuster.

Brecht, Bertolt
1965 The Caucasian Chalk Circle. New York: Grove Press.

Bursten, B. and R. D'Esopo
1965 "The obligation to remain sick." Archives of General Psychiatry 12:402–407.

Bushard, B. L.
1957 "The U.S. Army's mental hygiene consultation service." In Symposium on Preventive and Social Psychiatry. Washington: Walter Reed Army Institute of Research.

Butler, Samuel
1961   Erewhon. New York: Collier.

Butler, Willis P.
1969   "Cuba's revolutionary medicine." Ramparts 7 (March):6–14.

California Department of Public Health
1972   California State Plan for Hospitals. Berkeley: The Department.

Carlson, Clifford and Gary Athelson
1970   "The physician's assistant." Journal of the American Medical Association 214:1855–1861.

Carnoy, Judith
1970   "Kaiser: you pay your money and you take your chances." Ramparts 9 (November):27–31.

Cartwright, Ann
1964   Human Relations and Hospital Care. London: Routledge & Kegan Paul.

Chapman, C. B. and J. M. Talmadge
1971   "The evolution of the right to health concept in the United States." Pharos 34:30–51.

Cherry, Colin
1966   On Human Communication. Cambridge: MIT Press.

Children's Hospital Medical Center
1970   Family Health Care Program, case records. Boston, Mass., 02115.

Chomsky, Noam
1965   Aspects of the Theory of Syntax. Cambridge: MIT Press.

Cloward, Richard and Lloyd Ohlin
1960   Delinquency and Opportunity. New York: Free Press.

Coleman, J. V.
1967   "Social factors influencing the development and containment of psychiatric symptoms." In Mental Illness and Social Processes, ed. T. J. Scheff. New York: Harper & Row.

Colombo, T. J. et al.
1969   "The integration of an OEO health program into a prepaid comprehensive group practice plan." American Journal of Public Health 59:641–650.

Colombotos, John
1969   "Physicians and Medicare: a before-after study of the effects of legislation on attitudes." American Sociological Review 34:318–335.

Commonwealth of Massachusetts
1970   Public Assistance Policy Manual, Chapter IV, Section A, page 3, item 2. Massachusetts: Department of Public Welfare.

Connally, J. P. et al.
1966   "Physician and nurse—their interprofessional work in office and hospital ambulatory settings." New England Journal of Medicine 275:765–769.

Cronkhite, L. W. et al.
1971   "A health care system for Massachusetts." New England Journal of Medicine 284:240–243.

Crozier, Michel
1964   The Bureaucratic Phenomenon. Chicago: University of Chicago Press.

Cumming, Elaine
1968   Systems of Social Regulation. New York: Atherton.

Dahl, Robert
1957   "The concept of power." Behavioral Science 2:201–215.

Dahrendorf, Ralf
1959 Class and Class Conflict in Industrial Society. Stanford: Stanford University Press.

Daniels, Arlene Kaplan
1969 "The captive professional: bureaucratic limitations on the practice of military psychiatry." Journal of Health and Social Behavior 10:255–265.

Davis, Fred
1960 "Uncertainty in medical prognosis: clinical and functional." American Journal of Sociology 66:41–48.
1963 Passage Through Crisis. Indianapolis: Bobbs-Merrill.

Davis, M. S.
1968 "Variations in patients' compliance with doctors' advice: an empirical analysis of patterns of communication." American Journal of Public Health 58: 274–288.

Dodgen, J. C. and J. B. Brickman
1967 "The psychotherapy of maladjusted Marine recruits." Military Medicine 132: 913–916.

Dorsey, Joseph L.
1973 "The prepaid group practice plan in the education of future physicians." Medical Care 11:12–20.

Downs, Anthony
1967 Inside Bureaucracy. Boston: Little, Brown.

Dube, W. F. et al.
1971 "Study of U.S. medical school applicants, 1970–71." Journal of Medical Education 46:837–857.

Duff, R. S. and A. B. Hollingshead
1968 Sickness and Society. New York: Harper & Row.

Duhl, L. J.
1969 "Newark: community of chaos: a case study of the medical school controversy." Journal of Applied Behavioral Science 5:537–572.

Durkheim, Emile
1958 The Rules of Sociological Method. Glencoe, Ill.: Free Press.

Egbert, L. D. et al.
1964 "Reduction of postoperative pain by encouragement and instruction of patients." New England Journal of Medicine 270:825–827.

Ehrenreich, Barbara and John Ehrenreich
1969 "The big business of health." Liberation 14 (December):23–31.
1973 "Hospital workers: a case study in the 'new working class.' " Monthly Review 23:12–27.

Erikson, Kai T.
1957 "Patient role and social uncertainty—a dilemma of the mentally ill." Psychiatry 20:263–274.
1962 "Notes on the sociology of deviance." Social Problems 9:307–314.
1966 Wayward Puritans. New York: Wiley.

Fanon, Frantz
1967 "Medicine and colonialism." In A Dying Colonialism. New York: Grove.

Feifel, H.
1966 "Death." In Taboo Topics, ed. N. L. Farberow. New York: Atherton.

Fein, Rashi
1967 The Doctor Shortage. Washington: Brookings.
1970 Quoted in Daniel Schorr, Don't Get Sick in America. Nashville: Aurora.

Feldstein, Paul J.
1966   "Research on the demand for health services." Milbank Memorial Fund Quarterly 44:128–165.

Field, Mark
1953   "Structured strain in the role of the Soviet physician." American Journal of Sociology 58:493–502.
1957   Doctor and Patient in Soviet Russia. Cambridge: Harvard University Press.
1967   Soviet Socialized Medicine. New York: Free Press.

The Financing Workshop
1969   "The Blue Cross we bear." Health-PAC Bulletin, September, pages 2–6.

Fortune Magazine
1970   "Our ailing medical system." Fortune 81 (January):79 ff.
1972   "The Fortune directory of the 50 largest life-insurance companies." 85 (May): 212–213.

Fox, Renée C.
1957   "Training for uncertainty." In The Student-Physician, ed. R. K. Merton et al. Cambridge: Harvard University Press.
1959   Experiment Perilous. Glencoe, Ill.: Free Press.
1968   "Illness." In International Encyclopedia of the Social Sciences. New York: Macmillan and Free Press.
1970   "A sociological perspective on organ transplantation and hemodialysis." Annals of the New York Academy of Science 169:406–428.

Frake, C. O.
1961   "The diagnosis of disease among the Subanun of Mindanao." American Anthropologist 63:113–132.

Francis, V. et al.
1969   "Gaps in doctor-patient communication: patients' response to medical advice." New England Journal of Medicine 280:535–540.

Frank, D. A.
1970   "Hospitals and me don't take: a participant observation study of physically ill adolescents." Honors thesis, Department of Social Relations, Harvard University.

Fredericks, Marcel A. et al.
1971   "Physicians and poverty programs." Hospital Progress 52 (March):57–61.

Freidson, Eliot
1961   Patients' Views of Medical Practice. New York: Russell Sage.
1970a Profession of Medicine. New York: Dodd, Mead.
1970b Professional Dominance. New York: Atherton.

Freire, Paolo
1970   Pedagogy of the Oppressed. New York: Herder and Herder.

Friedman, Milton
1962   Capitalism and Freedom. Chicago: University of Chicago Press.

Fuchs, V. R.
1966   "The contribution of health services to the American economy." Milbank Memorial Fund Quarterly 44:65–101.

Gamson, William A.
1968   "Stable unrepresentation in American society." The American Behavioral Scientist 12:15–21.

Gans, Herbert
1972   "The positive functions of poverty." American Journal of Sociology 78:275–289.

Garceau, Oliver
1941   The Political Life of the American Medical Association. Cambridge: Harvard University Press.

Genet, Jean
1966 Miracle of the Rose. New York: Grove.

Glaser, Barney and Anselm Strauss
1965 Awareness of Dying. Chicago: Aldine.

Glaser, William A.
1970 Paying the Doctor. Baltimore: Johns Hopkins.

Goffman, Erving
1961 Asylums. Garden City, N.Y.: Doubleday.

Gordis, Leon and Milton Markowitz
1971 "Evaluation of the effectiveness of comprehensive and continuous pediatric care." Pediatrics 48:766–776.

Gordon, Gerald
1966 Role Theory and Illness. New Haven: College & University Press.

Gouldner, Alvin W.
1954 Patterns of Industrial Bureaucracy. New York: Free Press.
1970 The Coming Crisis of Western Sociology. New York: Basic Books.

Greenberg, I. G. and M. L. Rodburg
1971 "The role of prepaid group practice in relieving the medical care crisis." Harvard Law Review 84:887–1001.

Greenberg, Selig
1965 The Troubled Calling. New York: Macmillan.

Greenlick, M. R. et al.
1972 "Comparing the use of medical care services by a medically indigent and a general membership population in a comprehensive prepaid group practice program." Medical Care 10:187–200.

Griffiths, H. W.
1968 Instructions for Patients. Philadelphia: Saunders.

Guevara, Che
1968 "On revolutionary medicine." In Venceremos: The Speeches and Writings of Che Guevara, ed. John Gerassi. New York: Simon & Schuster.

Halberstam, M. J.
1971 "Liberal thought, radical theory and medical practice." New England Journal of Medicine 284:1180–1185.

Hapgood, David
1969 "The health professionals: cure or cause of the health crisis?" Washington Monthly 1 (June):60–73.

Hardin, Garrett
1968 "The tragedy of the commons." Science 162:1243–1248.
1972 Exploring New Ethics for Survival. New York: Viking.

Harper, Gordon
1969 "Ernesto Guevara, M.D.: physician—revolutionary physician—revolutionary." New England Journal of Medicine 281:1285–1289.

Harris, F. G. and R. W. Little
1957 "Military organizations and social psychiatry." In Symposium on Preventive and Social Psychiatry. Washington: Walter Reed Army Institute of Research.

Harris, Richard
1966 A Sacred Trust. New York: New American Library.

Harvard Medical School
1971 "Information and instructions concerning the National Internship and Residency Matching Program (NIRMP)." Mimeographed, Office of Student Affairs.

Health-PAC Bulletin
1969 "The Medicaid blues." September, page 6.
1972 "Columbus Hospital: 2 steps forward, one step back." October, page 24.

Health Policy Advisory Center
1970 The American Health Empire. New York: Random House.

Hiatt, H. H.
1971 "Medical care for Northbridge." New England Journal of Medicine 284:593–602.

Homans, George C.
1964 "Contemporary theory in sociology." In Handbook of Modern Sociology, ed. R. E. L. Faris. Chicago: Rand-McNally.

Horn, Joshua S.
1969 "Away With All Pests . . .": An English Surgeon in People's China. New York: Monthly Review Press.

Inkeles, Alex
1963 "Sociology and psychology." In Psychology: A Study of a Science, ed. S. Koch. New York: McGraw-Hill.

Israel, Joachim
1971 Alienation. Boston: Allyn and Bacon.

Janis, I. L.
1958 Psychological Stress: Psychoanalytic and Behavioral Studies of Surgical Patients. New York: Wiley.

John, Roy et al.
1971 "Public health care in Cuba." Social Policy 1 (5):41–46.

Kadish, Joseph and James Long
1970 "The training of physician's assistants: status and issues." Journal of the American Medical Association 212:1047–1051.

Karpinos, B. D.
1967 "Mental test failures." In The Draft, ed. Sol Tax. Chicago: University of Chicago Press.

Kasl, S. and S. Cobb
1966 "Health behavior, illness behavior and sick role behavior." Archives of Environmental Health 12:246–266, 531–541.

Kelman, Sander
1971 "Toward the political economy of medical care." Inquiry 8 (3):30–38.

Kennedy, Edward M.
1971 "Bill S.3—Introduction of a bill to create a national system of health security." Congressional Record, January 25, 1971, Sections 47, 87, 103.
1972 In Critical Condition. New York: Simon & Schuster.

Komaroff, A. L.
1971 "Regional medical programs in search of a mission." New England Journal of Medicine 284:758–764.

Koos, Earl
1967 The Health of Regionville. New York: Hafner.

Korsch, B. M. et al.
1968 "Gaps in doctor-patient communication: doctor-patient interaction and patient satisfaction." Pediatrics 42:855–871.

Korsch, B. M. and V. F. Negrete
1972 "Doctor-patient communication." Scientific American 227 (August):66–74.

Kosa, John et al., eds.
1969 Poverty and Health: A Sociological Analysis. Cambridge: Harvard University Press.

Kropotkin, Peter
1972a The Conquest of Bread. New York: New York University Press.
1972b Mutual Aid. New York: New York University Press.

Laing, R. D.
1969   The Divided Self. Baltimore: Penguin.
1972   The Politics of the Family. New York: Vintage.

Lasker, Judy
1971   "Health care delivery: an institutional perspective." Unpublished paper, Department of Sociology, Harvard University.

Lawton, Denis
1968   Social Class, Language and Education. London: Routledge & Kegan Paul.

Lenin, V. I.
1939   Imperialism. New York: International.

Lenski, Gerhard E.
1956   "Social participation and status crystallization." American Sociological Review 21:458–464.
1966   Power and Privilege. New York: McGraw-Hill.

Levy, Howard and Oliver Fein
1972   "Crippled H.I.P." Health-PAC Bulletin, October.

Lewis, Charles E. and R. S. Hassanein
1970   "Continuing medical education—an epidemiological evaluation." New England Journal of Medicine 282:254–259.

Lewis, C. E. and H. W. Keairnes
1970   "Controlling costs of medical care by expanding insurance coverage." New England Journal of Medicine 282:1405–1414.

Lewis, C. E. and B. A. Resnick
1967   "Nurse clinics and progressive ambulatory patient care." New England Journal of Medicine 277:1236–1241.

Lichtman, Richard
1971   "The political economy of medical care." In The Social Organization of Health, ed. Hans Peter Dreitzel. New York: Macmillan.

Lippmann, Walter
1962   "The underworld as a servant." In Organized Crime in America, ed. Gus Tyler. Ann Arbor: University of Michigan Press.

Little, R. W.
1956   "The 'sick soldier' and the medical ward officer." Human Organization 15: 22–24.

Lydston, G. F.
1911   "Malingering among criminals." Journal of Criminal Law and Criminology 2:386–388.

McGhee, A.
1961   The Patient's Attitude to Nursing Care. Edinburgh: Livingston.

Malinowski, Bronislaw
1926   "Anthropology." Encyclopedia Britannica, first supplementary volume. London: Encyclopedia Britannica Co., pages 132–133.
1939   "The group and the individual in functional analysis." American Journal of Sociology 44: 938–964.

Maloney, J. V.
1970   "A report on the role of economic motivation in the performance of medical school faculty." Surgery 68:1–19.

Mao Tse-tung
1961   "In Memory of Norman Bethune." In Selected Works, Vol. 2, p. 337. San Francisco: China Books.

Marmor, T. R.
1968   "Why Medicare helped raise doctors' fees." Trans-Action 5 (September): 14–19.

Marx, Karl
1906   Capital. Chicago: Kerr.
1963   Early Writings, ed. T. B. Bottomore. London: Watts.
1964   "Estranged labor." In Economic and Philosophic Manuscripts of 1844. New York: International.

Marx, Karl and Frederick Engels
1948   The Communist Manifesto. New York: International.
1968   "The Eighteenth Brumaire of Louis Bonaparte." In Selected Works, by Karl Marx and Frederick Engels. New York: International.

Maslow, Abraham
1963   "The need to know and the fear of knowing." Journal of General Psychology 68:111–125.

Massachusetts Department of Public Health
1972   "Certificate-of-need program." New England Journal of Medicine 287:307.

Mechanic, David
1959   "Illness and social disability: some problems in analysis." Pacific Sociological Review 2:37–41.
1962   "The concept of illness behavior." Journal of Chronic Diseases, 15:189–194.
1968   Medical Sociology: A Selective View. New York: Free Press.
1972   "Social psychologic factors in presentation of bodily complaints." New England Journal of Medicine 286:1132–1139.

Mechanic, David and Edmund Volkart
1960   "Illness behavior and medical diagnosis." Journal of Health and Human Behavior 1:86–94.
1961   "Stress, illness, and the sick role." American Sociological Review 26:51–58.

Medical Committee for Human Rights
1970   Delegation to observe Cuban medical system, personal communication.
1972   "Position paper on national health care." In Billions for Band-aids, ed. Tom Bodenheimer et al. San Francisco: The Committee.

Medical Defence Union and Royal College of Nursing
1961   "Memorandum on steps that might be taken to obviate the risk of an operation being performed on the wrong patient, side, limb or digit." London: Royal College of Nursing.

Melville, Herman
1952   White Jacket, or the World of a Man-of-War. New York: Grove Press.

Merrium, Arnold
1971   "The rise and decline of social insurance in America." Honor's Thesis, Department of the History of Science, Harvard University.

Merton, Robert K.
1968   Social Theory and Social Structure. New York: Free Press.

Michels, Robert
1962   Political Parties. New York: Free Press.

Miller, S. M. and Pamela Roby
1970   The Future of Inequality. New York: Basic Books.

Mills, C. Wright
1967   The Sociological Imagination. New York: Oxford.

Moore, Gordon T. et al.
1972   "Effect of a neighborhood health center on hospital emergency room use." Medical Care 10:240–247.

Moore, Thomas G., Jr., and Thomas Bodenheimer
1973   "Feelings about the Kaiser Foundation Health Plan on the part of Northern California carpenters and their families," duplicated, California Council for Health Plan Alternatives and Medical Committee for Human Rights.

Moore, W. E. and M. M. Tumin
1949   "Some social functions of ignorance." American Sociological Review 14: 787–795.

Nagel, Ernest
1961   The Structure of Science. New York: Harcourt, Brace & World.

National Intern and Residency Matching Program
1973   Results: Number of Interns/Residents Sought and Number Matched for Each Participating Hospital. Evanston, Ill.: The Program.

Navarro, Vincente
1972   "Health services in Cuba: an initial appraisal." New England Journal of Medicine 287:954–959.

Norman, Frank
1958   Bang to Rights. London: Secker & Warburg.

Oken, D.
1961   "What to tell cancer patients: a study of medical attitudes." Journal of the American Medical Association 175:1120–1128.

Olson, S. W.
1971   "Health insurance for the nation." New England Journal of Medicine 284: 525–533.

Parsons, Talcott
1951   The Social System. New York: Free Press.
1966   "On the concept of political power." In Class, Status, and Power, ed. Reinhard Bendix and S. M. Lipset. New York: Free Press.
1969   "Research with human subjects and the professional complex." Daedalus 98 (2):325–360.
1970   Social Structure and Personality. New York: Free Press.
1972   "Definitions of health and illness in the light of American values and social structure." In Patients, Physicians and Illness, ed. E. Gartly Jaco. New York: Free Press.

Parsons, Talcott and Renée C. Fox
1952   "Illness, therapy, and the modern urban American family." Journal of Social Issues 8:31–44.

Perrott, G. S. and J. C. Chase
1969   "The Federal Employees Health Benefits Program." Health and Welfare News, October.

Peterson, O. L. et al.
1956   "An analytical study of North Carolina general practice." Journal of Medical Education 31:1–165.

Piven, Frances Fox and Richard A. Cloward
1971   Regulating the Poor: The Functions of Public Welfare. New York: Vintage.

Pollack, Jerome
1968   "The role of Blue Cross and the insurance companies in insuring group practice." Bulletin of the New York Academy of Medicine 44:1342–1345.

Popper, Karl
1959   The Logic of Scientific Inquiry. New York: Basic Books.

Pratt, L. et al.
1957   "Physicians' views on the level of medical information among patients." American Journal of Public Health 47:1277–1283.

Radcliffe-Brown, A. R.
1935   "On the concept of function in social science." American Anthropologist 37: 395–396.
1948   The Andaman Islanders. Glencoe: Free Press.

Rayack, Elton
1967   Professional Power and American Medicine. Cleveland: World.

Reader, G. et al.
1957   "What patients expect from their doctors." Modern Hospital 89 (1):88–94.

Representatives of Cuban Ministry of Public Health
1969   Communications to meeting of World Health Organization, Boston.

Rice, Dorothy P. and Barbara S. Cooper
1970   "National health expenditures, 1929–68." Social Security Bulletin 33 (January):3–20.

Richards, V.
1971   "Surgical education with full-paying patients." American Journal of Surgery 121:217–218.

Robert, Howard O. and Emil C. Tasser
1970   "Duke University's physician's assistant program." Hospital Progress 51 (February):49–55.

Roemer, Milton I. et al.
1972   Health Insurance Effects. Ann Arbor: School of Public Health, University of Michigan.

Roghmann, K. J. et al.
1971   "Anticipated and actual effects of Medicaid on the medical-care pattern of children." New England Journal of Medicine 285:1053–1057.

Rosen, George
1958   A History of Public Health. New York: M. D. Publications.

Rosen, S. and A. Tesser
1970   "On reluctance to communicate undesirable information: the MUM effect." Sociometry 33:253–263.

Roth, Julius A.
1963   "Information and the control of treatment in tuberculosis hospitals." In The Hospital in Modern Society, ed. Eliot Freidson. Glencoe, Ill.: Free Press.

Sade, R. M.
1971   "Medical care as a right: a refutation." New England Journal of Medicine 285: 1288–1292.

Saunders, Lyle
1954   Cultural Differences and Medical Care. New York: Russell Sage.

Scheff, T. J.
1966   Being Mentally Ill. Chicago: Aldine.

Schneider, D. M.
1964   "Social dynamics of physical disability in Army basic training." In Personality in Nature, Society and Culture, ed. Clyde Kluckhohn et al. New York: Knopf.

Schwartz, Harry
1972   "H. I. P.'s troubles: Is the cure worse than. . . .?" New York Times (April 30).

Selznick, Philip
1966   TVA and the Grass Roots. New York: Harper.

Shaw, George Bernard
1963   "Preface on doctors," preface to The Doctor's Dilemma. In Complete Plays With Prefaces, Vol. 1. New York: Dodd, Mead.

Shiloh, Ailon
1968 "The interaction between the Middle Eastern and Western systems of medicine." Social Science and Medicine 2:235–248.

Shuval, Judith
1970 Social Functions of Medical Practice. San Francisco: Jossey-Bass.

Sidel, V. W.
1972 "The barefoot doctors of the People's Republic of China." New England Journal of Medicine 286:1292–1300.

Skipper, J. K. and R. C. Leonard
1968 "Children, stress, and hospitalization: a field experiment." Journal of Health and Social Behavior 9:275–287.

Skipper, J. K. and R. C. Leonard, eds.
1965 Social Interaction and Patient Care. Philadelphia: Lippincott.

Somers, Anne R., ed.
1971 The Kaiser-Permanente Medical Care Program. New York: Commonwealth Fund.

Somers, Herman M. and Anne R. Somers
1967 Medicare and the Hospitals: Issues and Prospects. Washington: Brookings Institute.

Sox, Harold C., Jr., Carol H. Sox, and Richard K. Tompkins
1973 "Training of physicians' assistants by a clinical algorithm system." New England Journal of Medicine 288:818–824.

Stanford University School of Medicine
1972 "Application to the Association of American Medical Colleges for assistance in the development of a health maintenance organization," duplicated.

Straus, Robert
1957 "The nature and status of medical sociology." American Sociological Review 22:200–204.

Strauss, Anselm
1972 "Medical ghettoes." In Where Medicine Fails, ed. A. Strauss. New Brunswick, N.J.: Trans-Action Books.

Sykes, G. M.
1958 The Society of Captives. Princeton, N. J.: Princeton University Press.

Szasz, Thomas S.
1961 The Myth of Mental Illness. New York: Harper and Row.
1963 Law, Liberty and Psychiatry. New York: Macmillan.
1967 "The psychiatrist as double agent." Trans-Action 4 (October):16–24.
1970 The Manufacture of Madness. New York: Harper & Row.
1972 "Voluntary mental hospitalization: an unacknowledged practice of medical fraud." New England Journal of Medicine 287:277–278.

Titmuss, R. M.
1963 Essays on "The Welfare State." London: Unwin.
1971 The Gift Relationship. New York: Vintage.

Tyler, Gus
1962 Organized Crime in America. Ann Arbor: University of Michigan.

United Nations
1972a Statistical Yearbook, 1971. New York: United Nations.
1972b Demographic Yearbook, 1971. New York: United Nations.

U. S. Army
1959 Medical Service Theater of Operations, Field Manual FM 8–10. Washington: Department of the Army.

U. S., Department of the Army
1967 Medical Service—Standards of Medical Fitness. Washington: The Department.
1969 Results of the Examinations of Youths for Military Service, 1968, supplement to Health of the Army. Washington: The Department.

U. S., Department of Commerce
1972 Statistical Abstracts of the United States: 1972. Washington: U. S. Government Printing Office.

U. S., Department of Labor
1972 National Survey of Professional, Administrative, Technical, and Clerical Pay. Washington: U. S. Government Printing Office.

U. S., House of Representatives
1971 H. R. 1, 92nd Congress, First Session.

U. S., Internal Revenue Service
1970 U. S. Income Tax Regulations. Chicago: Commerce Clearing House.

Vogel, E. F. and N.W. Bell
1968 "The emotionally disturbed child as the family scapegoat." In A Modern Introduction to the Family, ed. N. W. Bell and E. F. Vogel. New York: Free Press.

Waitzkin, Howard
1969 "Conceptions of the sick role, with special reference to a penal institution." Unpublished paper, Department of Social Relations, Harvard University.
1970 "Expansion of medical institutions into urban residential areas: aftermath of the Harvard strike." New England Journal of Medicine 282:1003–1007.
1971 "Review of Poverty and Health, edited by John Kosa et al." American Journal of Sociology 76:1173–1176.

Waterman, Barbara
1971 "Impressions of the Yugoslavian health system." Unpublished paper, Department of Social Relations, Harvard University.

Weber, Max
1958a "Bureaucracy." In From Max Weber: Essays in Sociology, ed. H. H. Gerth and C. W. Mills. New York: Galaxy.
1958b "Structures of power" and "Class, status, party." In From Max Weber: Essays in Sociology, ed. H. H. Gerth and C. W. Mills. New York: Galaxy.
1964 The Theory of Social and Economic Organizations. New York: Free Press.

Weed, L. L.
1969 Medical Records, Medical Education, and Patient Care. Cleveland: Case Western Reserve Press.

Weinberg, A. N.
1969 "Pathophysiology of respiratory tract infections." Mimeographed, Harvard Medical School.

Weinerman, E. R.
1968 "Problems and perspectives of group practice." Bulletin of the New York Academy of Medicine 44:1423–1434.
1969 Social Medicine in Eastern Europe. Cambridge: Harvard University Press.

White, L. P.
1969 "The self-image of the physician and the care of dying patients." Annals of the New York Academy of Science 164:822–831.

Whyte, W. F.
1943 "Social organization in the slums." American Journal of Sociology 8:34–39.
1958 Street Corner Society. Chicago: University of Chicago Press.

Williams, T. F. et al.
1967 "The clinical picture of diabetes control, studied in four settings." American Journal of Public Health 57:441–451.

Woodcock, George
1962 Anarchism. Cleveland: Meridian.

Suggested Readings

The authors especially recommend the following readings. For full citations, see the reference list.

The American Health Empire, by the Health Policy Advisory Center (1970), which is also available in paperback form, presents the first major radical critique of the American health system. Though lacking traditional academic documentation and somewhat rhetorical at times, the book is useful for anyone concerned with problems of power, financial structure, and change in health institutions. The *Health-PAC Bulletin* is a publication of the Center which provides current analyses of similar themes.

Bodenheimer et al. (1972) gives a somewhat more documented and up-dated radical critique. This short book is a collection of articles, with discussions of several specific problems in the health system. The book also contains the "national health plan" of the Medical Committee for Human Rights.

Horn (1969) and Guevara (1968) provide inspiring analyses of the political implications of revolutionary change in health systems.

Freidson's two major books (1970a, 1970b) give extremely useful sociological critiques of professional autonomy and dominance, as major problems inhibiting improvements in the American health system. Despite some weaknesses which we discuss in Section 2, Freidson's work represents one of the outstanding analyses of the institution of medicine in recent years.

Parson's classic work in medical sociology (1951), despite its many analytic and empirical problems, should not be overlooked by students of the American health system or of medical sociology more broadly.

Recent analyses of the political economy of health care represent an innovative critical approach which should be encouraged (Alford, 1972; Kelman, 1971; Lichtman, 1971).

THE BOBBS-MERRILL REPRINT SERIES

The authors recommend for supplementary reading the following related materials. Please fill out this form and mail.

Indicate the number of reprints desired

___ **Bernstein, Basil** 1964 "Elaborated and Restricted Codes: Their Social Origins and Some Consequences." Ethnography of Communication, pp. 55–69. **S-549**/66926 40¢

___ **Cloward, Richard A.** 1959 "Illegitimate Means, Anomie, and Deviant Behavior." American Sociological Review, pp. 164–175. **S-44**/66450 40¢

___ **Davis, Fred** 1956 "Definitions of Time and Recovery in Paralytic Polio Convalescence." American Journal of Sociology, pp. 582–587. **S-366**/66744 40¢

___ **Dentler, Robert A. and Kai T. Erikson** 1959 "The Functions of Deviance in Groups." Social Problems, pp. 98–107. **S-71**/66477 40¢

___ **Field, Mark G.** 1953 "Structured Strain in the Role of the Soviet Physician." American Journal of Society, pp. 493–502. **S-83**/66488 40¢

___ **Frake, Charles O.** 1961 "The Diagnosis of Disease Among the Subanun of Mindanao." American Anthropologist, pp. 113–132. **A-72**/64054 40¢

___ **Freidson, Eliot L.** 1960 "Client Control and Medical Practice." American Journal of Sociology, pp. 374–382. **S-87**/66492 40¢

___ **Goffman, Erving** 1956 "The Nature of Deference and Demeanor." American Anthropologist, pp. 473–502. **S-400**/66778 40¢

___ **Gouldner, Alvin** 1970 "Toward The Radical Reconstruction of Sociology." Social Problems. **S-703**/68721 40¢

___ **Hall, Oswald** 1946 "The Informal Organization of the Medical Profession." Canadian Journal of Economics and Political Science, pp. 30–44. **S-110**/66513 40¢

___ **Hollingshead, August B. and Frederick C. Redlich** 1953 "Social Stratification and Psychic Disorders." American Sociological Review, pp. 163–169. **S-120**/66524 40¢

Malinowski, Bronislaw 1939 "The Group and the Individual in Functional Analysis." American Journal of Sociology, pp. 938–964.
S-183/66582 40¢

Marx, Karl and Frederich Engels 1848 The Communist Manifesto. pp. 2–48. **S-455**/66833 60¢

Merton, Robert K. 1948 "The Bearing of Empirical Research upon the Development of Social Theory." American Sociological Review, pp. 505–515. **S-466**/66844 40¢

Michels, Robert O. 1927 "Some Reflections on the Sociological Character of Political Parties." American Political Science Review, pp. 753–772. **PS-202**/65682 40¢

Moore, Wilbert E. and Melvin M. Tumin 1949 "Some Social Functions of Ignorance." American Sociological Review, pp. 787–795.
S-205/66603 40¢

Parsons, Talcott and Renée Fox 1952 "Illness, Therapy, and the Modern Urban American Family." Journal of Social Issues, pp. 31–44.
S-221/66617 40¢

Pilisuk, Marc and Thomas Hayden 1965 "Is There a Military Industrial Complex Which Prevents Peace?: Consensus and Countervailing Power in Pluralistic Systems." Journal of Social Issues, pp. 67–117. **S-742**/68759 80¢

Radcliffe-Brown, A. R. 1935 "On the Concept of Function in Social Science." American Anthropologist, pp. 394–402.
S-227/66623 40¢

Roth, Julius 1957 "Ritual and Magic in the Control of Contagion." American Sociological Review, pp. 310–314. **S-492**/66870 40¢

The Bobbs-Merrill Company, Inc.
College Division
4300 West 62nd Street
Indianapolis, Indiana 46268

Instructors ordering for class use will receive *upon request* a complimentary desk copy of each title ordered in quantities of 10 or more. Refer to author and *complete* letter-number code when ordering reprints.

☐ Payment enclosed   ☐ Bill me (on orders for $5 or more only)

_____ Course number   _____ Expected enrollment

☐ For examination   ☐ Desk copy

Bill To_____

ADDRESS_____

CITY_____STATE_____ZIP_____

Ship To_____

ADDRESS_____

CITY_____STATE_____ZIP_____

Please send me _____ copies of the sociology reprint catalog.

Please send me related reprints catalogs in_____

_____

Any reseller is free to charge whatever price he wishes for our books.

For your convenience please use complete form when placing your order.